Keto for Seniors:

2 Manuscripts: Keto After 50 & Keto for Women Over 50, A Gentler Approach to Ketogenic Diet Including a Cookbook with Delicious Recipes for Weight Loss and Bone Health

Thomas Slow

Text Copyright © Thomas Slow

All rights reserved. No part of this guide may be reproduced in any form without permission in writing from the publisher except in the case of brief quotations embodied in critical articles or reviews.

Legal & Disclaimer

The information contained in this book and its contents is not designed to replace or take the place of any form of medical or professional advice; and is not meant to replace the need for independent medical, financial, legal or other professional advice or services, as may be required. The content and information in this book have been provided for educational and entertainment purposes only.

The content and information contained in this book have been compiled from sources deemed reliable, and it is accurate to the best of the Author's knowledge, information, and belief. However, the author cannot guarantee its accuracy and validity and cannot be held liable for any errors and/or omissions. Further, changes are periodically made to this book as and when needed. Where appropriate and/or necessary, you must consult a professional (including but not limited to your doctor, attorney, financial advisor or such other professional advisor) before using any of the suggested remedies, techniques, or information in this book.

Upon using the contents and information contained in this book, you agree to hold harmless the Author from and against any damages, costs, and expenses, including any legal fees potentially resulting from the application of any of the information provided by this book. This disclaimer applies to any loss, damages or injury caused by the use and application, whether directly or indirectly, of any advice or information presented, whether for breach of contract, tort, negligence, personal injury, criminal intent, or under any other cause of action.

You agree to accept all risks of using the information presented inside this book.

You agree that by continuing to read this book, where appropriate and/or necessary, you shall consult a professional (including but not limited to your doctor, attorney, or financial advisor or such other advisor as needed) before using any of the suggested remedies, techniques, or information in this book.

Table of Contents

KETO FOR SENIORS: 0
TABLE OF CONTENTS 3
KETO AFTER 50: 9
INTRODUCTION 10
CHAPTER 1: KETOGENIC DIET BASICS 12

HISTORY OF THE KETOGENIC DIET 12
HOW THE KETOGENIC DIET WORKS 13
HEALTH BENEFITS OF THE KETOGENIC DIET 15
   Brain Benefits 16
   Heart Disease 16
   Fight Cancer 17
   Improve Sleep and Energy Levels 18
   Decrease Inflammation 18
   Gastrointestinal and Gallbladder Health 19
   Improved Kidney Function 20
   Improved Women's Health 21
   Improved Endurance and Muscle Gain 22
   Weight Loss 23
   Increased Metabolic Health 23
TYPES OF FATS FOR KETOSIS 26
QUICK START GUIDE FOR THE KETOGENIC DIET 33
COMMON MISTAKES TO AVOID 36

CHAPTER 2: KETOGENIC DIET AFTER 50 40

AGING AND NUTRITIONAL NEEDS 40
KETOGENIC DIET CHANGES FOR AGING ADULTS 47
FOODS TO ENJOY 48
   Fats and Oils 48
   Protein 50
   Fruits and Vegetables 52
   Nuts and Seeds 53
   Dairy Products 54

Spices and Condiments *56*
Sweeteners *57*
Beverages *58*
Foods to Avoid 59
Grains *60*
Sugar *60*
Low-fat Foods *60*
Starch *60*
Fruits *61*
Macronutrients 101 61
Keto for Women Vs. Men 63
Reaching Ketosis 64
Signs You Are in Ketosis 66
How to Create a Meal Plan 68
Supplements for Success 70

CHAPTER 3: OVERCOMING THE KETO FLU 73

What Is the Keto Flu? 74
Signs & Symptoms of the Keto Flu 74
Causes of the Keto Flu 75
How to Get Over the Keto Flu 79
Preventing the Keto Flu 83

CHAPTER 4: BASIC FITNESS FOR THE KETOGENIC DIET 85

Ketogenic Diet Impact on Exercise Performance 86
What to Eat While Exercising on Keto 87
Cardio on Keto 88
Tips and Tricks for Maximizing Benefits 89
Intermittent Fasting 90
Types of Fasting *91*

CHAPTER 5: KETO RECIPES FOR BREAKFAST 93

Spicy Egg Poppers 94
Stuffed Breakfast Pepper 96
Keto Breakfast Cookies 98
Cream Cheese Breakfast Bombs 100
Cheesy Chive Omelet 102

CHAPTER 6: KETO RECIPES FOR LUNCH 104

- CREAMY CHICKEN SALAD 104
- SPICY KETO CHICKEN WINGS 107
- CILANTRO AND LIME CREAMED CHICKEN 109
- CHEESY HAM QUICHE 111
- LOADED CAULIFLOWER RICE 113

CHAPTER 7: KETO RECIPES FOR DINNER 115

- BUTTERY GARLIC STEAK 115
- BAKED LEMON SALMON 118
- ONE SHEET FAJITAS 120
- BALSAMIC CHICKEN 122
- CHEESY KETO MEATBALLS 124

CHAPTER 8: KETO SALAD RECIPES 126

- PESTO CHICKEN SALAD 126
- FRESH SUMMER SALAD 128
- KETO TACO SALAD 130
- MIXED VEGETABLE TUNA SALAD 132

CHAPTER 9: KETO RECIPES FOR SNACKS 135

- SWEET CINNAMON ROLL FAT BOMB 136
- SAUSAGE AND CHEESE PUFFS 138
- FROZEN BERRY BITES 140
- CREAM CHEESE AND HAM ROLLS 141
- KETO-FRIENDLY CRACKERS 142

CHAPTER 10: KETO RECIPES FOR DESSERT 144

- CHOCOLATE PEANUT BUTTER BOMBS 145
- KETO ICE CREAM 147
- CHEESECAKE FAT BOMBS 148
- LEMON BARS 150
- KETOGENIC COOKIE DOUGH 151

CONCLUSION 153

KETO FOR WOMEN OVER 50 .... **154**
INTRODUCTION **155**
CHAPTER 1: KETO – AN OVERVIEW **157**
- What is the Keto Diet? 157
- What is Ketosis? 159
- How is Insulin Affected by the Keto Diet? 160
- Positive Effects of the Keto Diet 162
- Negative Effects of Keto 164
- Keto Mistakes 165

CHAPTER 2: KETO FOR WOMEN OVER 50 .... **168**
- General Nutritional Needs for Women Over 50 168
- Gentler Approach to Keto for Women Over 50 170
- Tracking and Macros 172
- Fasting Over 50 175
- Keto Diet for Longevity 177
- Exercise for Women Over 50 in Support of Keto 178
- Tips and Tricks for Ketogenic Weight Loss 182

CHAPTER 3: KETO FOOD AND KETOSIS **187**
- Food Quality 187
- Foods to Eat 189
- Proteins 192
- Carbohydrates 196
- Nutritional Food List 202
- Spices and Sauces for Flavor 217
- What Foods to Avoid 223
- Keto Approved Sweeteners 225
- Keto on a Budget 228
- Keto Away From Home 230
- Keto at Restaurants 232

CHAPTER 4: WHAT ARE THE BEST FATS ON KETO?
.... **234**
- Types of Fat 235
- Omega-3, Omega-6, Omega-9 237
- Fat Bombs 239

CHAPTER 5: NEGATIVE MOMENTS IN KETO...........240
- KETO FLU 240
- CONSTIPATION 242
- DIARRHEA... 243
- INSOMNIA 244
- DIET PLATEAUS... 245
- CHOLESTEROL AND KETO... 246

CHAPTER 6: KETO RECIPES 249
- BREAKFAST 249
  - *Keto-Friendly Breakfast Tortilla* 249
  - *Breakfast Sandwich* 251
  - *Banana Nut Muffins* 253
- SMOOTHIES AND BEVERAGES 256
  - *Coconut Green Smoothie* 256
  - *Strawberry Smoothie* 257
  - *Keto Mojito*... 258
- SOUP 260
  - *Chicken and Riced Cauliflower Soup* 260
  - *Spicy Creamy Chicken Soup* 262
  - *Broccoli Cheese Soup* 264
- SAUCES AND DIPS... 266
  - *Tzatziki* 266
  - *Satay Sauce*... 267
  - *Thousand Island Salad Dressing* 269
  - *Hollandaise Sauce* 270
- SIDE DISHES 272
  - *Mexican Cauliflower Rice* 272
  - *Green Beans and Bacon* 274
  - *Baked Spaghetti Squash* 275
- SNACKS 277
  - *Taco Flavored Cheddar Crisps* 277
  - *Keto Seed Crispy Crackers* 278
- BEEF – PORK – CHICKEN 280
  - *Slow Cooker Chilli* 280
  - *Chicken Parmesan* 282
  - *Baked Un-BBQ Ribs* 284

FISH 286
   Salmon skewers 286
   Coconut Salmon with Napa Cabbage 288
   Keto Tuna Casserole 290
VEGETARIAN 292
   Cinnamon Crunch Cereal 292
   Broccoli Cheese Fritters 294
   Asian Noodle Salad 296
DESSERT 298
   Cocoa Brownies 298
   Chocolate Chip Cookies 301
   Keto Brown Butter Pralines 303

CONCLUSION **305**

Keto After 50:

The Ultimate Guide to Ketogenic Diet for Men and Women over 50 Including:
Cookbook with Mouthwatering Recipes to Accelerate Weight Loss and Reset Your Metabolism

Introduction

Congratulations on purchasing *Keto After 50: The Ultimate Guide to Ketogenic Diet for Men and Women Over 50,* and thank you for doing so!

Before I started the Ketogenic Diet, I honestly struggled with my health and my lifestyle. I had no idea that the foods I was eating on a daily basis were slowly making me sicker by the day. While other diets had failed time and time again, I finally came across the Ketogenic Diet just before it was too late!

I decided to write this book to help people share the same success that I have. Through the science-backed Ketogenic Diet, I have lost thirty pounds and have changed my life for the better. While other diets have failed me, I have been following this lifestyle for five years now and will never go back!

That is one of the best parts of the Ketogenic Diet. While other diets are strict and hard to follow, the Ketogenic Diet is fairly basic once you grasp the basic concepts. Within the chapters of this book, you will find everything you need to know about the diet, including some tips and tricks I have learned along the way!

During my health journey, I hit just about every bump along the way. I have fallen off the ketosis-wagon time and time again. I hope that by preparing yourself with this book beforehand, you can get straight to the health benefits this diet has to offer! Honestly, it is one of the best decisions I have ever made for myself!

After you get through the basics of the diet and why it works for individuals, such as myself, over 50 years of age, you will be handed some of the most delicious recipes I have ever come across! Whether you are looking for a meal for lunch or dinner, I have got you covered! Yes, I have even included some of my favorite snacks and desserts for you to try because they are allowed and also encouraged on your new diet!

I hope that by the end of this book, you will feel like a Ketogenic Diet expert. As I said earlier, it changed my life for the better, and with some hard work and determination, it can change yours as well. When you are ready, we will start from the beginning of the diet.

Chapter 1: Ketogenic Diet Basics

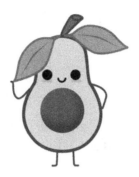

Before starting any diet, it is crucial you understand the history behind it. As you well know, there are many diets on the market in the modern age. The right question you need to ask for yourself is, Is the Ketogenic Diet right for you? Luckily for all of us, the Ketogenic Diet can help a wide range of individuals, whether you are young, older, or somewhere in between!

History of the Ketogenic Diet

The Ketogenic Diet first began in the 1920s and 30s. Initially, it was a popular therapy for individuals who had epilepsy. At the very beginning, the Ketogenic Diet was first developed to provide an alternative to fasting, which also worked well for epilepsy therapy.

While the diet did work for a while for these patients, it was eventually abandoned when modern medicine came around and was able to help a majority of patients with their symptoms. However, there were still approximately 30% of patients where the medication did not work, and the diet was re-introduced to help these individuals.

In 1921, it was an endocrinologist known as Rollin Woodyatt that was one of the first to notice the three water-soluble compounds that are produced in the liver when we are starved from carbohydrates. These three compounds are what we now know as ketone bodies. It was at this point, an individual from the Mayo Clinic known as Russel Wilder would call this "starvation from carbohydrates" as the Ketogenic Diet!

As the diet continues to grow in popularity, there is more research being performed on the Ketogenic Diet by the day! With science-backed evidence, you can follow the diet and know for a fact that it is going to work.

How the Ketogenic Diet Works

Welcome to your first Ketogenic Diet Science lesson! One of the best parts of the Ketogenic Diet is the fact that it is based around a natural process that your body already has! The key to success is fueling your body correctly instead of stuffing it with overly-processed junk. In this guide, you will learn everything you need to know from what to eat when to eat and how to get into the best shape of your life!

The first lesson you need to know is that our body has four primary fuels that we use. These include glucose, protein, free fatty acids, and ketones. Each one of these fuel sources are stored in different proportions in our bodies. Overall, the fuel that we use the most is stored as triglyceride in our adipose tissue, aka, FAT! The second most used source is protein and glucose, which are used depending upon the metabolic state of your body.

So, what determines what fuel to use and when? As you might have already guessed, the primary determinant is based upon carbohydrate availability. Additional factors that can affect fuel utilization include a full or empty liver glycogen level and the levels of certain enzymes. Overall, total energy equals glucose plus FFA.

Next, it is vital that you understand that the body has three different fuel storages that it taps into when you begin to lower your calories. These three different storage depots include protein, carbohydrates, and fats! Protein is essential in your diet because it can be converted into glucose in your liver and then used as energy. Carbohydrates are typically stored as glycogen and are placed in your liver and muscle. Fat, on the other hand, is generally stored as body fat, but we will get to that in a second.

When you are following a SAD diet or a Standard American Diet, ketones truly have a non-existent role when it comes to your energy production. However, as you begin a ketogenic diet, it will play a much more significant role, and here we introduce the fourth potential fuel source for your body! As you start to decrease the carbohydrate availability through diet, your body will automatically make the shift to using fat as your first fuel source.

Health Benefits of the Ketogenic Diet

As you can tell, there are some extremely complex biological processes behind the Ketogenic Diet. When you first start this diet out, you will want to consult with a doctor before you begin any changes. As far as any diet goes, it is crucial that you choose one that is going to benefit you rather than do more harm. For this reason, be sure to consult with a professional before you experiment on yourself.

With that in mind, why begin any diet if it isn't going to benefit you? Before you dive into the diet itself, let's learn all of the incredible ways that the Ketogenic Diet can help you. Whether you are looking to lose weight, gain energy, or improve brain function, the ketogenic diet may be just what you were searching for.

Brain Benefits

As you begin to change the fuel source for your body, this includes significant fuel sources for your brain as well. <u>Studies</u> have found that through the Ketogenic Diet, individuals were able to increase the stability of their neurons as well as the up-regulation of the mitochondrial enzymes and brain mitochondria.

With that in mind, scientists have been <u>studying</u> how a Ketogenic Diet may be able to benefit those who have Alzheimer's disease. It seems as though through diet, individuals have been able to enhance their memory as well as increase cognition. When this happens, a diet may be able to bring improvement to individuals with all different stages of dementia.

For those who do not need to worry about Parkinson's disease or Alzheimer's Disease, the Ketogenic Diet is also <u>beneficial</u> in increasing mental focus, clarity, and could potentially grant less frequent and less intense migraines. Generally, these conditions are related to altered brain chemistry and stable blood sugar levels, both helped by the Ketogenic Diet.

Heart Disease

Another major benefit that makes people take a look at the Ketogenic Diet is the downstream effects of the diet on blood glucose levels. As you begin to cut carbohydrates from your diet, it can help keep your blood glucose stable and low. By doing this, individuals have been able to keep their blood pressure in check and are also able to lower their triglyceride levels.

When people first begin a Ketogenic Diet, they feel that it is counterintuitive to eat a higher percentage of fat in order to lower the triglycerides, but the truth is, fat has had a bad rep this whole time! In fact, it is eating excessive carbohydrates, especially fructose, that is the culprit behind increasing triglycerides! The truth is, through this new diet, you will be able to raise your good cholesterol and lower your bad cholesterol.

Fight Cancer

When it comes to cancer, it is essential that you seek medical attention before you try to take your life into your own hands through diet. It is highly advised that you listen to your doctor's advice when it comes down to cancer treatment. However, there have been articles published based around cancer and the ketogenic diet.

In 2014, Dom D'Agostino's lab published an article based around ketones being able to decrease tumor cell viability in mice that had metastatic cancer. Within this article, it was found that, generally, cancer cells will express an abnormal metabolism that is characterized when glucose consumption is increased. When this happens, the genes begin to mutate, and the mitochondrial begins to malfunction. In the studies, it is found that cancer cells are unable to use ketone bodies as energy, therefore inhibiting the viability of the tumor cell in the first place!

Improve Sleep and Energy Levels

Unfortunately, many individuals underestimate how important sleep is. The good news is that after only four or five days on the ketogenic diet, many individuals have reported that they already begin to <u>benefit</u> from higher energy levels. On a scientific level, this may be due to the fact that through your new ketogenic diet, you will be stabilizing your insulin levels. As your body becomes stabilized, this will help provide you with a ready source of energy rather than experiencing the spikes and crashes.

As far as sleeping goes, the ketogenic diet affects sleep are still being studied. Right now, it seems as though through diet, individuals are able to decrease the time they spend in REM and increase slow-wave sleep patterns. It is believed that this is due to a <u>biochemical shift</u> in the brain as your body learned to use ketones as energy. Either way, you will be sleeping more in-depth and longer than before, granting you a fresh start to each day!

Decrease Inflammation

Inflammation is a strange defense mechanism used in the body to help the immune system recognize any damaged cells, pathogens, or irritants. Through inflammation, the body is able to identify these issues and begin the healing process. While this is beneficial for the most part, it, unfortunately, can persist longer than needed and will end up causing more harm than good.

If you have inflammation in your body, you may experience symptoms such as pain, redness, swelling, immobility, and sometimes even heat. But, these signs of inflammations only apply to the inflammations on the skin. Sometimes, inflammation can happen within our internal organs, and that is when we experience symptoms such as fever, abdominal pain, chest pain, mouth sores, and even fatigue.

<u>Studies</u> have found that the key player in inflammation, and the diseases associated with it, is suppressed BHB. Luckily through the ketogenic diet, BHB is one of the primary ketones you will be producing as you begin your new diet. This meaning that you will be able to help issues, including IBS, eczema, psoriasis, acne, and even arthritis, all through diet!

Gastrointestinal and Gallbladder Health

If you suffer from heartburn or acid reflux on a daily basis, you may want to take a good, hard look at your diet. Unfortunately, many sugary foods, nightshade vegetables, and grain-based foods are major culprits of both heartburn and acid reflux. With that in mind, it shouldn't come as a surprise that when you change your diet to include low-carb foods, these symptoms will disappear almost instantly. The reason you experience these issues is through an autoimmune response, bacterial issue, and inflammation caused by these foods in the first place.

Another benefit of the Ketogenic Diet will be the altering of the microbiome found in your gut. An individual known as Dr. Eric Westman found that through diet, individuals are able to significantly reduce health issues as they change their microbiome. In fact, he believes that when you take away carbohydrates, this can fix just about any gastrointestinal issues that affect a number of different people.

Along those same lines, research has also found that carbohydrates may be a significant culprit behind gallstones as well. As far as the Ketogenic Diet goes, it appears that when individuals consume a diet that is higher in fat, this can help keep the system running smoothly and will prevent gallstones from forming in the first place.

Improved Kidney Function

Another common issue among the health community is kidney stones. The most common cause of both gout and kidney stones is due to elevated levels of phosphorus, oxalate, calcium, and uric acid in the body. Unfortunately, this is often combined with obesity, dehydration, bad genetics, sugar consumption, and alcohol consumption.

Through the Ketogenic diet, individuals are able to lower their uric acid levels and help improve the health of their kidneys. It should be noted that while the ketogenic diet can help long-term, this diet does temporarily raise the uric acid levels within the body, especially if you are dehydrated. While it does <u>rise</u> as the ketone levels rise, the uric acid levels will lower in about four to six weeks.

Improved Women's Health

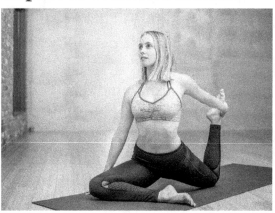

While the ketogenic diet is beneficial for both men and women, studies have shown that through diet, women may be able to stabilize their hormones and increase their fertility.

There was extensive research published in 2013 that looked at the key evidence linking ketogenic diets to enhancing fertility. It was also found that the Ketogenic Diet can treat PCOS (Polycystic Ovary Syndrome.) Through diet, individuals were able to eliminate or reduce symptoms of PCOS, including obesity, acne, and prolonged menstrual periods.

On a more general basis, it seems as though with this diet, individuals were able to keep their blood sugar levels low and stable. When this happens, it helps stabilize and equilibrate hormone levels, especially in women. Fortunately, this is a downstream benefit of the metabolic pathways that are related to insulin. Overall, individuals feel more balanced and stable than ever!

Improved Endurance and Muscle Gain

As we get older, we generally begin to lose the muscle mass we once had. As mentioned earlier, one of the main ketones you will begin producing as you begin the Ketogenic Diet is BHB. BHB is helpful in promoting muscle gain. When you combine the ketogenic diet with proper exercise, you will be increasing your health and muscle gain at the same time.

In addition to muscle gain, it is also believed that the diet can help improve endurance. Studies have found that athletes who switched to the diet and became fully fat-adapted showed significant improvements in both their mental and physical performances. Of course, this was compared to individuals who followed a typical diet that is rich in carbohydrates.

Weight Loss

Weight loss is one of the major reasons anyone begins a diet. Luckily through the ketogenic diet, there is substantial evidence that by eating the proper foods, you will be able to lose weight and preserve your muscle mass. In a related study, it was found that individuals who followed a ketogenic diet, compared to individuals on a low-calorie and low-fat diet were able to lose 2.2 times more weight! In addition, these people also improved their HDL cholesterol and Triglyceride levels.

The best part about losing weight on the Ketogenic diet is the fact that individuals are still able to lose fat without restricting their calories nor controlling their food intake. This is important to keep in mind when it comes down to sticking to any diet. When individuals hate the extra work of counting their calories, they are statistically more likely to return to their old eating habits. Later in this book, we will be going over the specifics of weight loss on the Ketogenic Diet.

Increased Metabolic Health

The last health benefit we will focus on in this chapter will be increased metabolic health. Metabolic syndrome is described as give common risk factors for heart disease, type 2 diabetes, and obesity. These include high blood sugar levels, low levels of HDL "good" cholesterol, high levels of LDL "bad" cholesterol, abdominal obesity, and high blood pressure. The good news is that many of these risk factors can be eliminated or improved through better lifestyle and nutritional changes.

An important factor behind these issues is insulin. Insulin plays a vital role as far as metabolic disease and diabetes go. Luckily, the Ketogenic Diet is very effective when it comes to lowering insulin levels for individuals who are prediabetic or have type 2 diabetes.
In one study, it was found that after only two weeks following the Ketogenic Diet, individuals were able to improve their insulin sensitivity by 75% and showed a blood sugar level drop from 7.5 mmol/l to a 6.2mmol/l! In another 16-week study, seven out of the 21 participants were able to stop their diabetic medication completely when they began the Ketogenic Diet.

As you can tell, the Ketogenic Diet can help a number of different people. While that is important to know, it is more important to understand how it works. The key to your success is going to be fat! While that may seem backward, what we are taught about fat is all backward! Yes, there are bad fats that we have to avoid, but good fat is going to be your new fuel source. Therefore, we will next learn the different types of fat you need to boost your success on the Ketogenic Diet.

Types of Fats for Ketosis

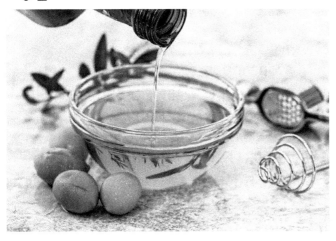

When you are following a Ketogenic Diet, about 70% of your calories will now be coming from fat sources. With that in mind, it can be hard figuring out which fats are healthy for you and which ones you should avoid. Below, you will learn the different types of fat you will be able to enjoy along with the keto-friendly sources you can find them in.

Good Fats

As a majority of fat is going to make up your new diet, it is important that you have a thorough understanding of the good fats that you will be able to enjoy.

The four main categories of fats that you will be picking from include saturated fats, polyunsaturated fats, monounsaturated fats, and naturally-occurring trans fats. Below, we will dive into each category to help give you a better idea of the fats you will want to keep an eye out for.

Saturated Fats

The most common misconception about fat circles around saturated fats. For years, this type of fat was believed to be harmful to the heart. In turn, the American Heart Association started the low-fat and fat-free craze in the 1970s. Luckily, recent studies have been debunking the claim that there is a link between disease and saturated fats. Instead, a balanced level of fat is now being <u>linked</u> to improved nutrition absorption, improved cognition, and balanced hormones.

One of the most popular types of saturated fat is medium-chain triglycerides. You probably know this more commonly as MCTs. MCTs can be found mainly in coconut oil but also is found in small amounts in palm oil and butter. The good news is that these saturated fats are easily digested by the body and get to the liver immediately for energy!

As you begin figuring out your diet, you will want to consider MCT oil. With this simple supplement, you can gain <u>benefits</u> such as boosting your immune system, suppressing your appetite, improving gut health, reducing the risk of heart disease, and even improving athletic performance. Saturated fat is also beneficial for enhancing your HDL and LDL cholesterol levels, maintaining bone density, and creating hormones such as testosterone and cortisol. Other good sources include:

- Cocoa Butter
- Heavy Cream
- Ghee
- Butter
- Red Meat
- Eggs

Monounsaturated Fats

The next type of fat we will be discussing are monounsaturated fats. Unlike with saturated fats, MUFAs have been known to be the healthy fat for a number of years now. MUFAs are linked to health benefits, such as increased insulin resistance and better cholesterol. This type of fat is also known to help lower blood pressure, lower an individual's risk for heart disease, and can even help reduce belly fat!

Luckily, MUFAs are found in a number of different healthy foods! Some of the more popular sources include:

- Avocados
- Avocado Oil
- Olive Oil
- Pecans
- Cashews
- Lard
- Bacon Fat

Polyunsaturated Fats

Here is when things can get a little tricky. When it comes to polyunsaturated fatty acids (PUFAs), it all comes down to how you use them. When polyunsaturated fats are heated, they form free radicals. Essentially, this means that this type of fat forms harmful compounds that can end up increasing your risk of cancer, cardiovascular disease, and inflammation. With that in mind, you will want to make sure that the sources of your PUFAs are cold and never used for cooking.

When appropriately used, PUFAs actually offer some great benefits. PUFAs provide you with essential nutrients of omega-3 and omega-6 fatty acids. Ideally, the radio of these should be around 1:1. On a standard western diet, the ratio of this is about 1:30. With that in mind, you will want to focus on PUFAs that are higher in omega-3s. Some of the <u>benefits</u> that come with proper levels of PUFAs include decreased risk of stroke, heart disease, autoimmune disorders, and inflammatory diseases. PUFAs also help <u>reduce</u> symptoms caused by depression and ADHD and improve overall mental health.

Some of the healthy forms of PUFAs will be:

- Nut Butter
- Nuts
- Chia Seeds
- Sesame Oil

- Fish Oil
- Fatty Fish
- Sardines
- Flax Oil
- Walnuts
- Olive Oil

Natural Trans Fats

As far as good and bad fats go, trans fats can get a little tricky. A mass majority of trans fats are going to fall under the "bad" category, as they are harmful and unhealthy, but here we are discussing naturally occurring trans fats. This type of trans fat is known as vaccenic acid. Some of the health benefits that come along with vaccenic acid include reduced risk of heart disease, diabetes, and obesity. Naturally occurring trans fat could possibly protect against cancer as well. Generally, this type of trans fat is going to be found in grass-fed meats and dairy fats.

Bad Fats

As you can tell, there are many different types of dietary fats that you will be able to enjoy on the Ketogenic Diet. With all of the good in mind, now it is time to learn the types of fat you will want to either eliminate or reduce drastically in your new diet. Bad fats will slow down your weight loss process and could have adverse health effects. Luckily, there is power behind knowledge, and you will know the good and the bad before you even begin.

Polyunsaturated Fats and Processed Trans Fats

When people refer to "bad" fat, they are talking about processed trans fats. Unfortunately, this type of fat makes up a majority of consumed fats and are incredibly damaging to one's health. Generally, these artificial trans fats are formed during the production of food, through the processing of the polyunsaturated fats. For this reason, you will want to choose PUFAs that have been unprocessed. As you will recall, heated PUFAs create harmful free radicals.

Some of the primary sources of trans fats come from hydrogenated oils that are found in fast food, crackers, cookies, margarine, and more. They are also found commonly in oils like canola, soybean, peanut, sunflower, and cottonseed. When this type of fat is consumed, it could increase your risk of certain cancers, heart disease, and your LDL levels. Trans fats also increase body fat and lead to unwanted weight gain. Overall, you will want to learn how to reduce this fat in your diet so you can benefit from the good fats.

Plant-based Fats

Later in this book, you will learn that there are several different types of the Ketogenic Diet. Some individuals choose to follow a Vegan Ketogenic Diet. Therefore, I feel it was important to include a section based around plant-based fats. It does become slightly more complicated, but there are definitely sources of fat out there that are plant-based.

1. Nuts
   The diet industry has gone back and forth whether nuts are healthy for us or not. Luckily, on the Ketogenic Diet, nuts are an excellent source of both protein and monounsaturated fats. Some of the better nuts for you to incorporate into your diet will be Brazil nuts, almonds, and walnuts.
2. Seeds
   Another common source of protein for you to consider will be seeds! Seeds are great because they can be sprinkled on anything from breads to sweets to salads! Seeds such as hemp seeds and chia seeds have an excellent source of omega-3 fatty acids, and sunflower seeds provide monounsaturated fats.
3. Avocados
   Avocados have been growing in popularity by the day! Avocados are packed with monounsaturated fats and can be very versatile when it comes to cooking. Whether you enjoy guacamole or chocolate mousse, there are many different ways to pack extra good fats into your diet.
4. Coconut Oil
   One of the more common ways to incorporate plant-based fats into your diet will be through coconut oil. Coconut oil offers delicious flavors, can handle high

temperatures, and offers those MCTs we discussed earlier.

5. Cacao Nibs
Yes, chocolate is now considered a health food! However, it is important to avoid the chocolate that is found in candy bars; that type of chocolate is full of sugar and bad for your health. It turns out that dark chocolate offers both monounsaturated fats and anti-oxidants! While, of course, it is essential to keep any fat in moderation, it is good to have on hand!

Quick Start Guide for the Ketogenic Diet

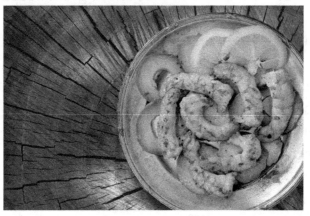

For those of you who are anxious to get started, there are a few basic rules you will want to follow when it comes to the Ketogenic Diet.

Good-bye Carbs

The golden rule to follow when starting your diet will be cutting the carbs! Later in the book, we will be going over macronutrients and how this pertains to your diet. For now, you will want to aim for your carb count to be 30 grams or under.

Eat Your Vegetables

As you learn to incorporate more fats into your diet, it should be kept in mind that fats are going to be higher in calories. If you are looking for weight loss on the Ketogenic Diet, you will want to make sure you are eating plenty of low-carb veggies to lower your overall caloric intake for the day. By doing this, you will be able to fill your plate and your stomach.

Make a Plan

When you first begin any diet, it can be hard to know where to start. Before starting the Ketogenic Diet, you will want to do some research to help you find low-carb meals for the week. Luckily within the chapters of this book, you will be provided with both recipes and a plan!

Trial and Error

On the Ketogenic Diet, there is going to be plenty of trial and error. The experimenting is half of the fun! While you will need to cut down on the carbs, there are plenty of other foods that you will be able to enjoy and are encouraged to try them all! Eventually, you will find your staples, and you will become a Ketogenic Pro!

Track Your Progress

This is honestly one of my favorite parts of starting the Ketogenic Diet. You may be reluctant to do this at first, but I promise that as the results begin rolling in, you will want to see how far you have come! Whether you take measurements, photos, or simply monitor your weight, you will want to continue doing this every three to four weeks. After a month alone, you may be pleasantly surprised just how far you have come.

Of course, there is much more to the Ketogenic Diet than this quick list, but it is an excellent place to get started. To further your knowledge on the subject, be sure to read the rest of this book!

Common Mistakes to Avoid

As you are well aware of at this point, there are some incredible benefits that come with the Ketogenic Diet. When you first start this diet, you are going to make a number of different mistakes. Whether you eat too many carbs, fall out of ketosis, or even just ditch your entire diet for the day, that is okay! What isn't okay is giving up this diet for good. Luckily because you are here, you will now learn some of the common mistakes people make on the Ketogenic Diet and how to avoid them in the first place!

Excess Protein
Excess protein intake is probably one of the biggest mistakes individuals make on this diet, especially when they are first getting started on the Ketogenic Diet. This is due to the fact that individuals give too much credit to the process of gluconeogenesis. You may be asking yourself, gluco-what? The method of gluconeogenesis is the process where your liver converts the protein you consume into blood glucose.

The key here is to realize that gluconeogenesis will only operate when it is on-demand, not when it is available. Essentially, this means that just because you ate a lot of protein in one day does not mean that it will automatically be converted into glucose. This process will only occur if your body needs glucose in the first place. So, while protein is going to be necessary on your diet, it should be consumed in moderation.

Excess Nuts and Dairy
As you learned earlier, dairy and nuts are both going to be significant sources of fats, but with that in mind, remember that these two foods are both calorie-dense. For this reason, it can become incredibly easy to overindulge on these foods, causing weight gain. Much like with protein, you can still enjoy these foods, but in moderation. If you feel dairy and nuts are trigger foods for you, you may want to try avoiding them for the first few weeks that you are following a Ketogenic Diet.

Adaption Time
While starting any diet, it is important not to expect results overnight. As you begin the Ketogenic Diet, you are going to be putting your body through some pretty profound changes. With such a significant difference, may come considerable struggles. Luckily, our bodies are pretty hardy when it comes to dealing with change and adapting to a different diet. It may seem frustrating at first, but you need to give your body time to adjust to your new diet. Remember that you are not just changing your diet; you are changing your overall fuel source! Give yourself some time, and the benefits will come before you know it.

Excess Carbohydrates
At this point, you are well aware that the Ketogenic Diet is based around limiting carbs. Unfortunately, this can be very tricky when you are first starting out. As you learn what you

can and cannot eat, you can expect to be in and out of ketosis fairly often. While this may be frustrating, you may want to take a closer look at your diet.

The key here is figuring out the maximum net carbs you can have in a day, depending on your activity level and metabolism. In the chapter to follow, we will be going more into depth on this subject. For general purposes, you will want to stay below 20 net carbs in a day to help you stay in ketosis. Once you become adapted to your new diet, you will learn precisely what your personal limit is and will excel from that point.

Snacking

In general, it is a pretty common habit to snack throughout the day. For some, this is to cure anxiety, and for others, its due to pure boredom! Snacking is also included in a number of different leisure activities, from dining out with friends to simply watching a movie.

If you are looking to lose weight on the Ketogenic Diet, you may want to limit your snacking. No matter what diet you follow, weight loss is equal to burning more calories than you consume. This rule is no different on your new diet.

Dehydration and Electrolytes

In the third chapter of this book, we will be tackling the dreaded Keto Flu. When you are first starting out, you will want to make sure you are staying hydrated and getting in enough electrolytes. The ketogenic diet has a dietetic effect, and when you lose water, you lose electrolytes. The three electrolytes you will want to focus on include magnesium, potassium, and sodium. Some of the best sources of potassium will be salmon, broccoli, spinach, and avocado. As long as you keep water and electrolytes consumption up, it will help you drastically while dealing with the symptoms of the Keto Flu.

Mindset
Finally, the most prominent mistake people make it not having the right mindset. If you are negative and miserable about your new diet, there is no way that you are going to stick with it! Instead, try your best to have a winner's mindset. This meaning that you start the diet off with clear goals and a reason behind your why. As you begin, ask yourself what is motivating you to begin this diet in the first place. What is going to drive you? Who are you doing this for? When you want to succeed at this diet more than anything else in the world, that is where you will find your success.

Now that you have a thorough understanding of Ketogenic Basics, it is time to learn how the Ketogenic Diet can help those of us who are over the age of 50! Yes, we are getting older, but life isn't over yet! There are still plenty of reasons to boost our health and perhaps live even better than when we were younger. If that sounds good to you, let's dive right into the next chapter.

Chapter 2: Ketogenic Diet After 50

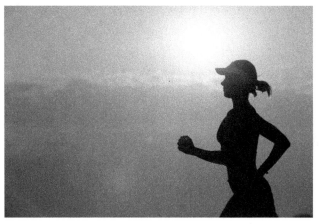

At any age, proper nutrition is incredibly important, but as we age, our bodies are going through some major changes. To help with these changes, it will be essential to make certain adjustments to our routines and nutrition. The vital factor to remember is that it is never too late to start taking care of yourself. When you neglect your health after the age of fifty, the effects may become more noticeable than ever before. So, how exactly does age affect our nutritional needs?

Aging and Nutritional Needs

As we age, you can expect a number of different changes to happen in your body, including thinner skin, loss of muscle, and less stomach acid. When these things happen, this can, unfortunately, make you more prone to nutrient deficiencies and overall quality of life. This is where the Ketogenic Diet comes in handy! By eating a variety of foods and incorporating the proper supplements, you will be able to meet your nutrient needs with no issues! Below, you will find some of the effects of aging and how to help the issue.

Less Calories- More Nutrients
On a general basis, an individual's daily calorie count will depend on a number of factors, including activity level, muscle mass, weight, and height. As for us older adults, we will need to begin lowering the number of calories we take in, in order to maintain or lose weight. Generally, older adults tend to exercise and move less compared to younger individuals.

While consuming fewer calories, it is important to continue getting higher levels of nutrients. For this reason, it is highly suggested to consume a variety of foods such as low-carb vegetables and lean meats to help get the proper nutrients and fight against any nutrient deficiencies. The nutrients you will want to focus on include vitamin B12, calcium, and vitamin D, Magnesium, Potassium, Omega-3 fatty acids, and Iron.

Benefits of Fiber
While many people do not like to discuss this, constipation is a prevalent health issue for individuals over the age of 50. In fact, women over the age of 65 are two to three times more likely to experience constipation! This may be due to

the fact that people over the age of 50 generally move less and are more likely to be taking a medication that has constipation as an unfortunate side effect.

To help relieve constipation, you will want to make sure you are getting enough fiber. When you eat more fiber, it is able to pass through your gut, undigested, and help regulate bowel movements and form stool. As an added benefit, high-fiber diets may also be able to prevent diverticular disease. Diverticular disease is a condition where small pouches build along the wall of the colon and become inflamed.

Focus on Protein
In the chapter above, you learned that it is important not to focus on protein, but it will be essential to find a balance on your new diet. As we age, it is very common to lose both strength and muscle. In fact, on average, an adult will lose anywhere between 3-8% of their muscle mass per decade after the age of 30. When we lose muscle mass, it could lead to poor health, fractures, and weakness among an elderly population. By eating more protein, you can help fight sarcopenia and maintain your muscle mass.

Vitamin B12
As mentioned earlier, keeping up with proper nutrients is going to be vital for your health. One of the vitamins you will want to focus on is Vitamin B12. This is a water-soluble vitamin that is in charge of making red blood cells and keeping your brain healthy. Unfortunately, it is estimated

that anywhere from 1—30% of individuals over the age of 50 have a lowered ability to absorb this vitamin from their diet.

One of the main reasons individuals over the age of 50 have difficulty absorbing vitamin B12 may be due to the fact that they have reduced stomach acid reduction. Vitamin B12 is bound to proteins. In order for your body to use this vitamin, the stomach acid separates it from the protein and becomes absorbed. To benefit your new diet, you will want to consider taking a supplement of vitamin B12 or consuming foods that are fortified with the vitamin.

Vitamin D and Calcium

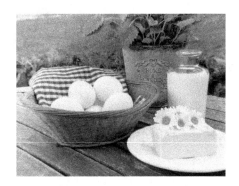

When it comes to bone health, calcium and vitamin D are going to be very important. While calcium is in charge of maintaining and building healthy bones, it depends on vitamin D to help the body absorb the calcium in the first place! Unfortunately, adults have a harder time absorbing calcium in their diets. This may be due to the fact that the gut absorbs less calcium as we age. However, the main culprit of a reduction in calcium is typically due to a vitamin D deficiency. As you can tell, they work hand in hand!

The reason we may experience a vitamin D deficiency is due to thinning skin. Generally, our body makes vitamin D from the cholesterol in the skin when it is exposed to sunlight. As the skin becomes thinner, it reduces the ability to make vitamin D and, in turn, reduces the ability to get enough calcium. When these two things happen, it increases the risk of fractures and bone loss.

To help counter this aging effect, you will want to make sure you are getting enough vitamin D and calcium in your diet. Some accessible sources will be dairy products, leafy vegetables, and dark greens. As far as Vitamin D goes, you will want to include a variety of fish or even a Vitamin D supplement such as cod liver oil.

Dehydration
On the Ketogenic Diet or not, staying hydrated is important at any age. In fact, water makes up about 60% of our bodies! Whether you are 20,30, or 50, the body still continually loses water through urine and sweat. As we age, it makes us more prone to dehydration.

When we become dehydrated, the water detects the thirst through receptors found all throughout the body and the brain. As we age, the receptors become less sensitive, making it hard to distinguish the thirst in the first place. On top of this, our kidneys are there to help converse water, but they also lose function with age.

Unfortunately, the consequences of dehydration are pretty harsh for the older population. When you are dehydrated long-term, this could reduce your ability to absorb medication and could worsen any medical condition. For this reason, it will be vital you keep up with your intake of water. I suggest trying a water challenge with friends and family or try having a glass of water with each meal you have.

Appetite
One of the last topics we will tackle on the subject of aging it the decrease in appetite. While this may seem like a benefit, a lack of eating could lead to a number of different nutritional deficiencies and unwanted weight loss. Poor appetite is most commonly linked to a heightened risk of death and overall poor health.

It is believed that some of the significant factors behind appetite loss could be due to changes in smell, taste, and hormones. Generally, older adults who have lower levels of hunger have higher levels of fullness hormones. When this happens, it causes individuals to be less hungry overall. As we age, the changes in smell and taste can also make food seem less appealing.

If you find this happens to you, you may want to establish a healthy habit of snacking. When you snack, try to reach for keto-friendly foods such as eggs, yogurt, and almonds to help put the nutrients back into your diet. If you are aware of this issue, it is something you can get a grasp on before it becomes a real problem.

Ketogenic Diet Changes for Aging Adults

As far as aging and nutrition go, it all comes down to a proper diet to help fuel you. The good news is that keto-friendly foods generally offer higher nutrition per calorie. This is vital as you already know that your basal metabolic rate is going to drop as you get older. Remember, the key here is to take in fewer calories but the same or more amount of nutrients! When you eat foods that are fighting disease and supporting your health, this will help you enjoy your golden years to the fullest.

The central concept you will want to promote for your new diet is to avoid empty calories. Empty calories generally come from foods that are high in sugars or lack nutrients, to begin with. You may have been able to live off junk food in your 20s, but you can kiss those days goodbye. Now, it is time to fill your plate with nutrient-dense foods.

No matter what your age is, it is never a bad idea to improve your health through diet. It is never too late to begin, and the sooner you start, the sooner you will feel better! The Ketogenic diet is meant for longevity. At this prime age, you will want to stop with the fad diets. They may work for a while, but it isn't worth doing if you aren't going to stick with the diet. Through the Ketogenic diet, you will be able to support your immunity, blood sugar levels, and put yourself at a healthier weight. If that all sounds good to you, let's take a look at what you can and cannot eat while following the Ketogenic Diet.

Foods to Enjoy

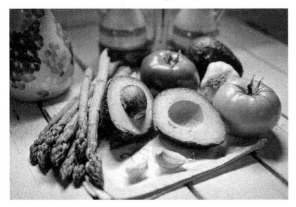

While starting a new diet can seem challenging enough, it is even harder when you are not sure what you can and cannot eat. Luckily, you will now find a comprehensive list of foods you will be able to enjoy while following a Ketogenic Diet. As you will soon find out, there is a wide variety of foods you will be able o enjoy, even if you are losing your beloved carbs.

Fats and Oils

As you already know, fats are now going to make up a majority of your calories in a day. The good news is that there a number of different ways to incorporate fats into your diet, whether you want to consume them as a dressing, sauce, or part of any meal!

When you are choosing fats for your diet, remember that eating the wrong type of fat can be dangerous for your health. As a quick recap, you will want to eat foods that have saturated, monounsaturated, and polyunsaturated fats while avoiding processed trans fats. This can be easily accomplished whether you are cooking with coconut oil, lard, or even tallow.

Another factor on the Ketogenic Diet to keep in mind will be balancing your omega 3 fatty acids and your omega 6 fatty acids. As you will recall from earlier, these are found in food sources such as shellfish, trout, tuna, and even salmon. These essential fatty acids are necessary for your health, but it is important to find that balance. Below, you will find a thorough list of foods that will provide the best sources of fats for your diet.

- MCT Oil
- Macadamia Oil
- Avocado Oil
- Coconut Oil
- Coconut Butter
- Ghee
- Butter
- Brazil Nuts
- Avocados
- Lard
- Fatty Fish
- Non-hydrogenated Animal Fat

- Egg Yolks
- Tallow
- Mayonnaise
- Cocoa Butter
- Olive Oil

Protein

When it comes to protein on the Ketogenic Diet, you will want to try your best to keep your portions in moderation. As you shop around for your protein sources, your best bet will be choosing protein that has been grass-fed and pasture-raised. By doing this, you will be able to minimize the intake of steroid hormones and bacteria.

As far as red meat goes, you pretty much can't go wrong! There are some cured meats and sausages that have added ingredients, but it is easy enough to avoid these. Instead, stick with fattier cuts of steak such a ribeye or fatty ratios of ground beef. Just remember that when you are incorporating protein into your diet, too much protein could kick you out of ketosis.

In order to balance the protein in your meals, you can pair them with a fatty sauce or side dish. Some of the best sources of proteins include:

- Nut Butters
  When you shop for nut butter, be sure that they are unsweetened and natural. Generally, you will want to

stick with macadamia or almond butter instead of peanut butter.
- Pork
There are many different types of pork for you to enjoy from ham, tenderloin, pork chops, pork loin, or even ground pork. When picking out pork, be sure to avoid added sugars and get the fattiest cuts possible.
- Beef
Beef is excellent to include on the Ketogenic Diet because it is incredibly versatile. When picking out beef, try to get fattier cuts of stew meat, roasts, steak, and ground beef.
- Eggs
Another excellent source of protein is going to come from whole eggs. These are great to have on hand because you can enjoy them in a number of different ways, from scrambled, poached, boiled, or even fried. When shopping for eggs, try to find them free-range.
- Shellfish & Fish
Finally, seafood is going to be an excellent source of protein for you. When shopping for fish, you will want to lean toward a selection that has been wild-caught. Look for fattier fish such as tuna, trout, snapper, salmon, mackerel, flounder, cod, and even catfish. As far as seafood goes, you can enjoy squid, mussels, scallops, crab, lobster, and even clams!

Fruits and Vegetables

Up until this point, you have probably learned that a balanced diet incorporates plenty of fruits and vegetables. While these are important for a balanced diet, some vegetables are high in sugar and low in nutrition. On the Ketogenic Diet, you will be consuming vegetables that are low in carbohydrates but still high in nutrients.

To stay on the safe side of vegetable selection, the secret to shopping will be sticking with vegetables that are grown above ground. Generally, these vegetables will be green, dark, and leafy. As you shop for your vegetables, you will want to opt for organic when possible, to help avoid pesticide residue. If you do find a vegetable that is grown below ground, this can still be enjoyed but in moderation. Below, you will find some low-carb vegetables for you to try.

- Spinach
- Baby Bella Mushrooms
- Green Bell Peppers
- Green Beans
- Romaine Lettuce
- Cabbage
- Cauliflower
- Broccoli
- Yellow Onion

As far as fruits go, these will generally be nonexistent on the Ketogenic Diet. Unfortunately, fruits typically have a higher carb count and are high in natural sugars. If you still crave some fruit, you can enjoy a limited amount of berries such as blueberries, blackberries, and raspberries. For cooking, you can also enjoy a limited amount of fresh lime and lemon juice.

Nuts and Seeds

Nuts are great to have on hand because they are an excellent source of fats, but remember to keep these in moderation because the carb count can add up quickly. You may also want to consider roasting the seeds and nuts to remove any anti-nutrients before enjoying it. Either way, raw nuts are great when you are looking to add texture or flavor to any meal. Nuts are also great for a quick snack.

As you choose your nuts, you will want to select from the following:

- Low Carb Nuts
  Some fatty, low carb nuts you will want to consider for your diet will be pecans, brazil nuts, and macadamia nuts. These are great to add a supplement of fat to your diet
- Moderate Carb Nuts
  Next, we have the fatty, moderate carb nuts. These include pine nuts, peanuts, hazelnuts, almonds, and walnuts. These can be added for flavor and texture but should be enjoyed in moderation.
- High Carb Nuts

The nuts you will want to avoid on the Ketogenic Diet will be cashews and pistachios. These are very high in carbohydrates and can easily kick you out of ketosis.

Dairy Products

As you begin the Ketogenic Diet, you will want a majority of your meals to come from fats, vegetables, and proteins. With that in mind, it is perfectly okay to enjoy dairy products in moderation. In general, you will want to make sure these products are organic or even raw. Unfortunately, dairy products that have been highly processed can contain anywhere from two to three times the amount of carbohydrates compared to the organic version. With that in mind, you will also want to choose products that are full fat. Some popular products include:

- Mayonnaise
- Hard Cheese
- Soft Cheese
- Whipping Cream
- Greek Yogurt

If you are looking to lose weight on the diet, it should be noted that some people have experienced slower weight loss when they ate too many dairy products. While it is okay to enjoy your share of cheese, you will want to keep dairy products in moderation. If you notice a slow down or plateau in your weight loss journey, cutting dairy would be a smart move to see if that is the culprit.

Cooking Flours

As you will find in a number of different recipes, cooking flours are going to be important to have on hand. Luckily, there are plenty of seed and nut flours for you to try out instead of regular flour. With that in mind, it will still be vital that you eat these in moderation.

Once you have become more comfortable with the Ketogenic Diet, you will learn how to combine multiple flours to get a better texture while baking. As you combine flowers, this can help you lower your net carbs if you are baking your own foods. You will want to keep in mind that these different flours do act in different ways. As an example, if you are cooking with coconut flour, you will want to use half the amount you would if you were using almond flour. Some of the more popular baking flours include:

- Flaxseed Meal
- Chia Seed Meal
- Coconut Flour
- Almond Flour
- Unsweetened Coconut

Spices and Condiments

Surprisingly enough, sauces and seasonings can be a very tricky part of the Ketogenic Diet. While many individuals freely use spices to add flavor to their meals, this is a sure way to add carbohydrates and processed ingredients without even knowing it!

While spices do have carbs in them, you will want to make sure you are counting them along the way. With that in mind, it should be noted that most of the pre-made spice mixes have added sugar. For this reason, you will want to make sure that you read any nutrition labels before you use or purchase an item. Below, you will find a list of common spices people still incorporate on their Ketogenic Diet.

- Pepper
- Sea Salt
- Thyme
- Rosemary
- Parsley
- Cilantro
- Oregano
- Cumin
- Basil
- Cinnamon
- Cayenne Pepper
- Chili Powder

When it comes to condiments and sauces, there seems to be a gray area on the Ketogenic Diet. If you want to be strict, you will want to avoid condiments and sauces as much as you can. Unfortunately, many of the pre-made condiments and sauces have added sweeteners or sugars that aren't keto-friendly. However, you can still make your own versions and avoid the excess carbs and sugars.

If you are desperate you can use some of the following in moderation:

- Ranch Dressing
- Yellow Mustard
- Low-sugar Ketchup
- Sriracha
- Vinaigrette Dressing
- Mayonnaise
- Soy Sauce
- Hot Sauce
- Horseradish
- Relish
- Sauerkraut

Sweeteners

When you first begin the Ketogenic Diet, it may be a good idea to stay away from sweet foods. By doing this, it can help keep your cravings to a minimum and can boost your success on the diet. However, if you genuinely need something sweet, it is better to have keto-friendly options to choose from.

As you begin searching for keto-friendly sweeteners, you will want to try to find one that is a liquid version. By doing this, you can avoid binders such as maltodextrin and dextrose that are higher in carbohydrates. Luckily, there are several sweeteners on the market that have a low glycemic impact. Some of the more popular sweeteners include:

- Stevia
- Monk Fruit
- Sucralose
- Erythritol

Beverages

Last but not least, we have keto-friendly beverages! As you learned earlier, the ketogenic diet has a natural diuretic effect. If you are just starting the diet, dehydration is a very common symptom to experience. On average, you will want to try your best to drink upward toward a gallon of water per day.

While water is important, it can become quite dull if it is the only liquid you are drinking. Another popular beverage people enjoy on the Ketogenic Diet is tea or Ketoproof coffee. Ketoproof coffee is excellent to have on hand to give you a boost of fat in the morning. Some other popular beverage choices include:

- Water, Water, and More Water!
- Broth
- Coffee
- Tea
- Almond Milk
- Coconut Milk

Foods to Avoid

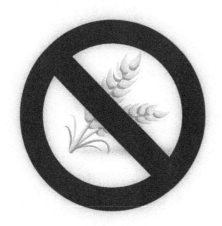

With a thorough understanding of the foods that you get to enjoy on the Ketogenic diet, it will be pretty easy to understand the foods that you will want to eliminate or avoid. If you are still unsure about any food items, it is probably safe to assume that they are not keto-friendly. While we want to focus on the positives of the Keto-genic diet, below you will find a list of foods you should avoid when you can.

Grains

This should be pretty much a given as you begin the Ketogenic Diet. Any wheat products such as beer, corn, rice, cakes, cereal, pasta, or bread need to be avoided on the Keto diet. It does not matter if it is made from quinoa, buckwheat, barley, rye, or wheat; these products are all going to be way too high in carbs.

Sugar

Much like with carbohydrates, you will want to avoid foods that are high in sugar. Typically, this means anything from ice cream, chocolate, candy, juice, soda, and even sports drinks. If it is processed and sweet, throw it out!

Low-fat Foods

As a society, we have been brainwashed to believe that low-fat foods are good for us! Unfortunately, these foods often have higher sugar and carb counts compared to the full-fat version. If you see low-fat on a package, it is best to leave it at the store.

Starch

While some vegetables are going to be tempting, it is best to stick with the list of approved vegetables in the section above. Some vegetables, such as potatoes and yams, are going to be too high in carbohydrates for the Ketogenic Diet. You will also want to avoid products like muesli and oats as well.

Fruits

Finally, you will want to avoid large fruits as well as you begin your diet. Anything from apples to bananas and oranges is going to be high in sugar and unnecessary for your diet. As mentioned earlier, you will still be able to consume berries in moderation.

As you can tell, there are plenty of foods that you will be able to enjoy on the Ketogenic Diet. While it will take quite a bit of trial and error, you will eventually find the foods that you truly enjoy, and you can make them staples in your daily diet.

Next on our list, it is time to learn about macronutrients. This is a vital lesson for anyone because your goals will be based on your macros, especially when you are trying to find your sweet spot for carbohydrates. When you are ready, let's move onto our next lesson.

Macronutrients 101

Whether you are looking to gain, lose, or maintain your weight, it will be important to understand what macronutrients are when starting a Ketogenic Diet. As you may already know, you will need to consume fewer calories when you are trying to lose weight and eat more if you are looking to gain weight. While it will take some time to figure out what your body needs, you will eventually find the sweet spot to achieve optimal health.

Macronutrients

You have probably heard of macronutrients before, but what are they exactly? Macronutrients are an organic or chemical compound that are consumed to give us the nutritional value and energy we need in order to survive. The macronutrients include proteins, carbohydrates, and fats.

- 1g of Carbs= 4 Calories
- 1g of Fat=9 Calories
- 1g of Protein=4 Calories

Fats

The first macronutrient we will discuss is fats. As you already know, there are unsaturated and saturated fats. This nutrient is essential because Vitamins K, E, D, and A can only be consumed in this form. On the Ketogenic Diet, around 70% of your calories will be coming from fat.

Protein

Next, we have Protein. Protein can be composed of several different types of amino acids and are the "building blocks" of the human body. Interestingly enough. Nine out of the twenty amino acids cannot be made by the human body, which is why it needs to be supplemented into the diet.

While protein is essential for just about everyone, it is especially important for individuals who plan on staying physically active. Protein is responsible for building new muscle tissue and repairing other tissues. While there is a significant debate on how much protein people need, you can use the general rule of thumb to eat one gram of protein per pound of body weight.

Carbohydrates
On the Ketogenic Diet, you will not have to pay much attention to carbohydrates because they are going to make up such a small part of your diet. It should be noted that there are two general categories of carbohydrates: Complex and Simple.

Simple carbohydrates are sugar molecules that can be digested quickly for an energy boost while complex carbs come from whole-food plants and contain a higher amount of fiber, minerals, and vitamins. When you do eat carbs, these will be the ones that you will want to reach for.

If you wish to calculate the macros to reach your personal goals, I suggest using a calculator online to find your magic numbers. With that in mind, remember that it will be vital that you keep your carb count under 20g in a day. If you are not in ketosis, there is no reason to be following the Ketogenic Diet.

Keto for Women Vs. Men

The truth is, there is a wide variety of people who can benefit from the Ketogenic Diet, whether they are young, old, man, or woman, but the Ketogenic Diet has been known to be especially beneficial for women due to their different hormones and conditions. This diet can be especially beneficial for women who are:

- Lacking results on other diets
- Binge on carbohydrates
- Planning on getting pregnant
- Want a healthy pregnancy
- Struggling with irregular periods
- Struggling with sex hormones
- Going through menopause

Reaching Ketosis

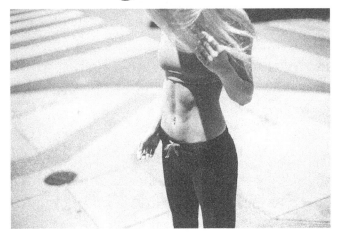

While you are following the Ketogenic Diet, being in Ketosis is going to be the key to your success. Ketosis is a natural state of your metabolic process. Once you have the ability to reach ketosis, this is when your body is going to begin burning the fat you have been storing instead of glucose.

When this process begins, there will be acids that will begin building up in your blood that are known as ketones. Luckily, ketones leave the body in your urine, but it will be important to keep track of the ketones in your body, as they can reach somewhat dangerous levels.

As a beginner, what you may not realize is that achieving ketosis is not as easy as it sounds. Below, you will find some ways to help you get into ketosis and stay there for the most benefit on your new diet!

1. Reduce Carbohydrate Intake
   The first step you are going to take on your new diet is reducing the number of carbohydrates in your diet. When you significantly reduce this number, it will force the body to use fat as energy rather than sugar. As noted earlier, the initial goal should be 20 grams per day or even less, if possible.
2. Increase Healthy Fat
   As you learn how to reduce the number of carbs in your diet, you will want to replace those calories with healthy fats. Remember that your diet is now going to be 70% fat, but it needs to be the right type of fat. Some healthy sources to start out with will be avocados, olive oil, and coconut oil!
3. Test Your Levels

After you have been following the diet for a few days, you will want to keep a close eye on your ketone levels. The best way to do this is by monitoring your levels with a test. Some of the popular versions include blood tests, breath tests, and urine tests. Each one of these are readily available at the store and should be taken on a daily basis. When you have an exact number, this could help you track what is kicking you out of ketosis.

4. Intermittent Fasting

    A prevalent practice on the Ketogenic Diet is intermittent fasting. While there are several ways to fast, you should speak with your doctor before completing a fast. In controlled cases, you should only fast for a period of ten to fifteen hours. When you go without food for a period of time, this could help put you into ketosis.

5. Physical Exercise

    If all else fails, you can always attempt increasing your physical activity. When you exercise, this will help deplete the glycogen stores you already have in your body. In most cases, these stores would be replenished with carbs, but on the Ketogenic Diet, your body will have no choice but to make the switch.

Signs You Are in Ketosis

As your body begins to undergo the biological adaption of ketosis, this will automatically trigger the reduction of your insulin levels and will increase your fat breakdowns. However, it can be hard to know if you are in ketosis or not. Luckily, there are several signs and symptoms that can tell you whether you are in ketosis or not!

Bad Breath
One of the most common symptoms that are reported on the Ketogenic Diet is bad breath! Bad breath is generally caused by elevated ketone levels, specifically the acetone that is exiting your body through breath and urine.

While this may be not so ideal for your social life, it is an excellent sign that you have reached ketosis! To help resolve this issue, you will want to consider sugar-free gum or just brushing your teeth a few more times a day.

Appetite Suppression
Another side effect of ketosis is appetite suppression. Many individuals have reported that they have decreased hunger while following their new diet. It is believed that this may be due to the increased vegetables and proteins, keeping you fuller for a more extended amount of time! It is possible that ketones also may affect the brain and reduce appetite.

Weight Loss
While following the Ketogenic Diet, you can expect weight loss, even in the first week! While, of course, this is primarily the water and carbs that have been stored in your body, it is just the beginning! Luckily, the Keto diet is known for both long-term and short-term weight loss.

Increased Ketones

As mentioned earlier, you will want to keep track of your ketones. The most reliable method of measuring these ketones is going to be using a blood meter, but you can also use a breath analyzer or urine strip. No matter which method you choose, you will notice an increase in ketones when your body is in ketosis.

Short Term Fatigue

A well-known side effect of the Ketogenic Diet is short-term fatigue. Remember that you are going to be switching the way your body runs, so this is an entirely natural side effect. As you probably expect, any switch you make is not going to happen overnight. In general, it takes people anywhere from seven to thirty days before they reach full ketosis. During this time, you will most likely experience some less than ideal side effects known as the Keto-Flu; we will cover everything you need to know about that in the next chapter. You will want to pay close attention here!

How to Create a Meal Plan

While building your knowledge of the Ketogenic Diet is important, it is just as important to come up with a plan for yourself! When you take the time to make a plan, it leaves less room for failure. As you learn how to follow a meal plan, you will never find yourself with an empty kitchen or, worse, a kitchen with temptations!

Luckily for you, it is easy enough to make your own meal plans, even if you have no idea what you are doing! If you are a true beginner, I suggest only planning one or two meals. As you become more comfortable with your diet and the foods you will be able to enjoy, you can build from that point.

Breakfast
The morning can be a tough time for people, especially when you are trying to get ready and have breakfast at the same time! When you have breakfast prepped already, it will make your life a million times earlier.
For breakfast, you will want to take some of the breakfast options provided them and batch cook them for the week! That way, all you will have to do is decide what you want for breakfast the night before, and you will be set for the morning.

Lunch or Dinner
As far as lunch goes, there is never any reason to go wild and crazy with your choices. All you need is a simple formula to help you create a balanced meal for yourself. The key here is to eat healthily but provide yourself with enough variety to help avoid any boredom. To create a balanced meal, choose one of each from the following list.

- Meat & Cooking Method
- Vegetable & Cooking Method
- Sauce

As long as your kitchen is stocked, you should be able to throw together a keto-friendly meal whenever you need it. Plus, if you make extra for dinner, there is your lunch for the next day! Remember to work smarter, never harder.

Snacks and Dessert
For weight loss purposes, remember that it is a better idea to leave the snacking and sweets behind. But if you are a busy person who is always on the run, it is better to carry snacks with you rather than cheat on your diet because you are in a pinch. Some excellent choices to stock up on could be:
- Pork Rinds
- Meat Sticks
- Dark Chocolate
- Low-carb Nuts

Just like that, you will be prepared for anything that comes your way!

Supplements for Success

When you are first starting the Ketogenic Diet, I suggest trying it for a few weeks on your own. It is going to take some extra effort, but it is absolutely something you can do naturally. If you need a little boost, there are some supplements on the market that can help ease the transition.

Alpha Lipoic Acid and Chromium

If you have issues with your insulin levels, Chromium and r-ALA may be able to help you out. While these two supplements claim to be insulin "mimickers," they actually help increase your sensitivity to insulin to help lower your insulin levels and heighten the glucagon. When this happens, you will get into ketosis quicker.

Hydroxymethylbutyrate (HMB)
This is a popular ketogenic supplement known as BHB salt. It is used as a supplement to minimize the period before you get into ketosis, aka The Keto Flu. HMB is an exogenous ketone, meaning you will be putting synthetic ketone fuel into your body before it naturally makes the change itself. By doing this, it will make the transition time easier.

Carnitine
You probably know this supplement as Acetyl L-Carnitine. This is a popular supplement to use as an energy booster. It seems now that L-Carnitine is actually needed to help boost the formation of ketones in the liver. When you take this supplement, it can help shift your metabolism from glycogen to ketones.

MCT Oil
When you reach ketosis, MCT Oil can be extremely beneficial in keeping you there. This oil has high-quality fats that can give you a quick boost when you need it in your diet. While this doesn't help make your transition more manageable, it will help once you are in ketosis.

Keto Multivitamin

For any people starting a strict kept diet, it can become challenging to get all of your essential fiber, minerals, and vitamins. For this reason, you may want to consider a quality multivitamin. This will help provide you with minerals that are all lost as you transition into ketosis. Either way, you will want to consider taking a supplement that provides you with electrolytes to help you out during the transition process.

Fish Oil

Finally, you will want to consider a supplement of fish oil. Remember that you will need to balance your omega-3s and omega-6s. While Americans generally get twenty times the amount of omega-6 fats they need, a fish oil or cod liver oil will be able to help you create that balance.

While supplements can be beneficial in some cases, they are not necessary. As mentioned earlier, you should give yourself a chance to follow this diet naturally. When you learn how to balance your plate and get your macros just right, you will be able to get into a stay in ketosis with no issue.

Now that you have learned the basics of the Ketogenic Diet, it is time to move onto the next chapter. I want to make sure that you pay close attention here because the Keto-Flu is no joke. It is something that we all go through, but with the tips and tricks provided in the next chapter, you will be able to get through it much easier than I did the first time!

Chapter 3: Overcoming the Keto Flu

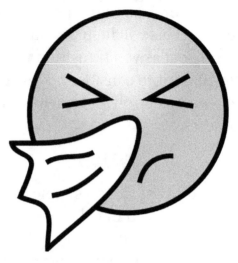

When you first begin the Ketogenic Diet, you are most likely anticipating all of the benefits people mention. While those changes will come at some point, you should be aware of the dreaded Keto Flu. Unfortunately, many people do not anticipate for this metabolic change, and they are unable to push through the potential side effects.

With that in mind, you will want to remember that the Keto flu is only going to be temporary! The fly is most prevalent when the body is attempting to transition into the new, ketogenic state. As soon as your body learns how to be fat-adapted, the symptoms will disappear before you know it!

The first step in tackling the Keto flu is going to be knowing what you are going up against. Luckily, with this book as your handy guide, you will be able to get through the flu with as much grace as possible. You could potentially feel awful, but if you can see the light at the end, you can get through anything. Let's start this chapter off by learning what the Keto flu is.

What Is the Keto Flu?

As you probably could have already guessed, the Keto flu is fairly related to the regular flu. The Keto flu comes about because your metabolism is trying to adjust to running on your new form of energy, fat. This is going to be a drastic change for your body, especially because, for the majority of your life, it has been running off glucose or carbohydrates for energy!

When you begin reducing your carb intake, this is going to begin depleting the glucose stores in your body. This switch can be tough on your body, and from here, you will begin to experience the flu-like symptoms. If you have ever had the flu before, you already know that it is not a great feeling.

Signs & Symptoms of the Keto Flu

So, what can you expect from this infamous Keto Flu? Some of the more common symptoms include:

- Low Energy Levels
- Sugar Cravings
- Lack of Focus
- Inability to Concentrate
- Irritability

- Heart Palpitations
- Insomnia
- Muscle Cramps
- Muscle Soreness
- Constipation
- Diarrhea
- Confusion
- Dizziness
- Nausea
- Stomach Pain
- Overall Brain Fog

If you are starting the Ketogenic Diet for the first time and are nervously awaiting the Keto-Flu, the symptoms listed above will generally start up around the first day or two of your diet. It should be noted that the length and strength of the symptoms are going to vary depending on the person. In fact, some people are lucky enough to skip the Keto flu altogether! Either way, you can rest assured that the symptoms will only last two weeks, at most. The sooner your body becomes fat-adapted, the better you will feel.

Causes of the Keto Flu

As you expand your knowledge of the Ketogenic Diet, you should be aware that there are four main causes of the keto flu. We will go over each source in detail below to help you lessen the blow of the flu in the first place.

Keto Adaption

Keto adaption is going to be one of the main culprits behind the Keto Flu. The body is incredibly complex and has two primary processes for energy. This includes glycolysis, which is burning glucose for energy and beta-oxidation, which is burning fat for energy. As your body adjusts, you will be switching from one process to the other. This switch is called your metabolic flexibility.

What many people don't realize is that genetics play a major role in our metabolic flexibility. If your metabolic flexibility is low, you are more likely to experience the symptoms of the keto flu. For this reason, some people handle the energy switch easier than others.

Carbohydrate Withdrawal
When you first make the switch to the Ketogenic Diet, you can expect a number of symptoms like cravings for sugar, irritability, and mood swings. There are <u>studies</u> that suggest that our brain is affected by sugar, similar to the way that it is affected by drugs such as cocaine or heroin. When we eat sugar, it releases the "feel good," hormone, dopamine. If you are not getting your "fix," your body is going to protest.

For this reason, when you begin to reduce the number of carbs in your diet, you can expect some of these symptoms. If your diet is currently heavy in refined carbs, sugars, and processed foods, you may have it worse off than others. While this doesn't mean you should jump off the Keto wagon instantly, you should anticipate the flu before it happens.

Lack of Micronutrients
People who first begin the Ketogenic Diet may have a hard time finding the proper balance when it comes to their macronutrients and their micronutrients. I understand that

it is difficult enough learning what you can and cannot eat, but these micronutrients are going to be important when it comes to your health.

As you begin the Ketogenic Diet, you already know that you are going to be cutting out a large number of grains, fruits, and vegetables. In order to make up for this, you will need to make sure you are eating a proper amount of keto-friendly foods that will still help you get your micronutrients in. Some of the best foods you can incorporate will be:

- Olive Oil
- Coconut Butter
- Fatty-cut Meat
- Seeds
- Nuts
- Fish
- Asparagus
- Spinach
- Eggplant
- Full-fat dairy

If you find yourself unable to get your micronutrients in, you may want to consider a supplement. Whether it is a multivitamin or a micronutrient powder, you will want to make sure that the item is free from additives, fillers, and sugars. This way, you won't have to worry about non-keto ingredients kicking you out of ketosis.

Electrolyte Imbalance
Last, but definitely not least, we have the electrolyte imbalance. When you begin to make the change of decreasing the number of high carb foods in your diet, you

can expect your body to begin losing water at an extremely fast pace.

This happens because the glucose that is stored in your body is bound to anywhere from 2-3 grams of water. As your body begins to adapt, your cells are going to use up the stored glycogen, meaning that the water weight you have been holding onto is going to get flushed out.

When all of this water is flushed out of your system, it is easy to become dehydrated and suffer from an imbalance of electrolytes. Once you become dehydrated, you may experience normal symptoms such as fatigue, headaches, and muscle pain. You will continue to feel this way until you balance your system out again.

For this reason, it will be vital that you are replacing the water and minerals that you are losing during this adaption period. The important minerals you will want to consider include potassium, magnesium, and sodium. By increasing your intake of these minerals, it can help ease your transition period.

The good news is that you will not feel like this forever! These symptoms are only temporary and will reduce as you learn how to put your body into ketosis properly. The even better news is that you can help get rid of the keto flu faster than you thought! Below, you will find some of my favorite tips and tricks of getting rid of the keto flu and jumping into the benefits of the Ketogenic Diet.

How to Get Over the Keto Flu

The anticipation of getting the keto flu can seem overwhelming, but the good news is that you are going to be able to help yourself. The reason people suffer from the keto flu for so long is that they have no idea what is happening to their body! Most people assume that they have to deal with the bad symptoms to get to the benefits of the diet. The truth is, these signs and symptoms from your body are like a cry for help! You don't just feel like junk for no reason! You will want to take the time to listen to your body and see how you can help yourself.

With that in mind, there are several steps you can take to help get you through the keto flu. Below, you will find some of my best tips to help you get over the keto flu and into ketosis with as little misery as possible.

Drink Up and Stay Hydrated
The number one tip I can give you as you begin the ketogenic diet is to stay hydrated! Even if you think that you are drinking enough water, you probably aren't. Staying hydrated should be your top priority as you begin the transition period into ketosis.

As mentioned earlier, water loss is to be expected as you begin your new diet, so these liquids need to be replenished simultaneously. The more often you are drinking, the easier the transition will come. You will see how much drinking water is going to reduce those awful symptoms of nausea, fatigue, and even those wicked headaches.

The best trick up my sleeve to help you drink more water through the day is to keep it in sight! I have a reusable water bottle that is by my side all day long. If you have a visual cue, it acts as an instant reminder to drink more water. I also suggest drinking a majority of the water during the day because it isn't so fun getting up to use the bathroom ten times a night.

Think Electrolytes
While we are on the topic of getting enough water, you will want to keep in mind that balancing your electrolytes is going to be just as important.

Before the ketogenic diet, many people don't have to worry about their electrolytes unless they are highly athletic. As mentioned earlier, your body is about to flush a mass majority of your water weight and electrolytes out of your system during this transition period. With that in mind, it should be noted that people lose electrolytes differently. The good news is that there are several ways for you to mitigate this imbalance.

The first tip I have for you will be increasing your sodium intake! When you increase the sodium in your diet, this could help counterbalance the water loss that is happening in your body. With that in mind, you will want to consider a supplement of Himalayan pink salt rather than the table salt most people have in their house. You would be amazed at the additives found in simple table salt!

Next, you will want to consider eating keto-friendly foods that are rich in potassium. Potassium is in charge of energy production, body temperature, bladder control, heartbeat regulation, and even muscle cramping. If you find yourself having symptoms in any of these areas, you probably need to up your potassium levels. Some of the best sources of this will be pumpkin seeds, mushrooms, and delicious avocado!

Another mineral you will want to make sure you are getting is magnesium. When people have low magnesium levels, this could lead to insulin resistance and depression. To ensure you are getting enough of this micronutrient in your diet, you will want to include food sources like dark chocolate, macadamia nuts, pumpkin seeds, and salmon.

On the Ketogenic Diet, calcium is also going to be important. While most people think that calcium is only important for bone health, it is also vital for your cardiovascular health, muscle contractions, and blood clotting. For this reason, it is a good idea to consume calcium-rich foods like salmon, chia seeds, and leafy greens.

Increase Fats
When your body begins switching over to its new source of energy, you are going to want to make sure that you are providing it with enough fat! Unfortunately, many people are shy about their fat intake when they are first starting their diet because we have been told our whole life that fat is bad! Now that your body is no longer using carbohydrates

and sugar as energy, you will need to give your body what it needs!

As you increase your fat consumption while reducing your carb consumption, this will help push your body into using the fat as energy. If you need, you can always supplement with MCT oil to help increase your ketone levels. It is also a good idea to up your fat source and includes foods such as:

- Coconut Oil
- Cacao Butter
- Olive Oil
- Heavy Cream
- Ghee
- Grass-fed Butter
- Avocado Oil
- Bacon Fat
- Walnuts
- Chia Seeds
- Pecans
- Flaxseed
- Fatty Fish
- Sesame Seeds

Work it Out

The next way to help get you over the keto flu will be exercise! This can be hard for some people, especially if they are unable to work through the symptoms provided by the keto flu in the first place. For this reason, I highly suggest light exercise anywhere from two to three times a week.

As you begin moving your body, this will help the switch drastically. As soon as you get over the keto flu, you will be able to resume your normal exercise routine. If you are first starting out, I highly suggest low-intensity exercises. You can try something like yoga, swimming, or even a light walk.

With exercise, you will be able to boost your metabolic flexibility and get over the keto flu before you even know it.

Exogenous Ketones
If none of the above work for you, you can always consider exogenous ketones. While your body is attempting to make the switch into ketosis, your body may not be producing enough ketones. For this reason, you may want to add ketone salts or exogenous ketones into your morning routine. By providing your body with what it needs, you can provide your system with ketones before you have even burned through the glycogen stores.

Preventing the Keto Flu

While it is beneficial knowing how to get over the keto flu, it is even better knowing how you can prevent it in the first place! If you are like everyone else in the world, you simply do not have the time to get sick! The good news is that there are some ways that you may be able to skip the keto flu altogether.

Follow the Diet
One of the main reasons beginners fall into the Keto-Flu is due to the fact that they are not following the diet the way they are supposed to! The keto diet best when you are getting the proper micronutrients as well as the right number of macronutrients.

The key to getting to your results is learning how to balance your nutritional needs. Yes, you could hit your macronutrients eating nothing but cottage cheese, but this is a sure way to dive right into the Keto flu. While it is going to be important for you to avoid carbohydrates, you will want to learn how to incorporate plenty of vegetables and seeds to help you get the nutrients you need.

The Power of Sleep
Unfortunately, many people are unaware of how important sleep is for the body. When you are first starting the Ketogenic diet, you will want to get at least seven to eight hours of sleep at night. When you are sleeping more, this could help reduce the fatigue and stress that comes along with the metabolism switch. If you struggle with sleep at night, you may want to consider a couple of power naps during the day!

Supplement
If you feel nothing is working, you can always consider taking a supplement or two. While, of course, you can get everything you need from a balanced diet, some people prefer the ease of a supplement. In the chapter above, you will find a list of some of my favorite supplements to give a try when you need a boost.

Chapter 4: Basic Fitness for the Ketogenic Diet

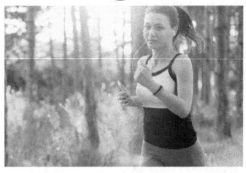

Whether you are following a Ketogenic Diet or not, exercise is almost always beneficial. As you begin to change your diet, you will experience rapid health changes already, but with exercise, you will be able to take your health to a whole new level!

As mentioned earlier, it can be slightly difficult to begin exercise routines when your body is first learning how to get into ketosis. When you are first starting out, you will want to try your best to keep things light but still get your body moving. The question is, how do exercise and the Ketogenic Diet relate?

Ketogenic Diet Impact on Exercise Performance

When you first start the Ketogenic Diet, you will be restricting your carbs. As this process happens, you will be limiting the sugar access for your muscle cells. Once your muscles lack this sugar, they will begin to lose their ability to function at high intensities. For this purpose, high intensities are any activity that can last more than ten seconds.

Due to this process, any activity in the muscle that requires max effort for anywhere from ten seconds to 120 seconds requires sugar. The thing about fat and ketones is that it cannot and never will stand-in for sugar. It is after two minutes of exercise that your body knows how to shift its metabolic pathways and starts burning fat and ketones.

For this reason, you will want to avoid any extreme exercise Some popular examples include

- HIIT (High-Intensity Interval Training)
- Sports such as Lacrosse and Soccer
- Swimming
- Lifting Weights

What to Eat While Exercising on Keto

If you do plan on exercising while on a Ketogenic Diet, it is going to be vital that you get your macronutrients down. Of course, what you eat is going to depend on your goals. Are you looking to gain muscle or lose weight?

Muscle Gain
If you are looking to gain muscle on the Ketogenic Diet, you are going to want to eat more keto-friendly foods. On average, you will want to consider eating anywhere from 250-500 calories extra per day. By doing this, you will be increasing your body weight as well.

Next, most of the calories should be coming from fat. Most athletes put protein as their most important macro, but that isn't true on the Ketogenic Diet. Inf act, your protein intake should only be around one gram of protein per lean body mass that you have. On that note, is carb restriction is impairing your exercise, you may want to consider intermittent fasting.

Fat Loss
When it comes to fat loss, remember that slow loss is still a loss. As you first begin your new diet, you are going to notice weight loss without any exercise, anyway. Generally, you

will want to cut down on calories anywhere between 250 and 500 calories. Weight loss comes down to calorie deficit. If you are overweight or obese, you may want to consider a higher calorie deficit.

If you still fail to lose weight after several weeks, consider lower fat intake. That seems counterproductive on the Ketogenic Diet; however, fat is still high in calories. You can still make a majority of your meal's fat-based, but enjoy them in smaller portions.

Cardio on Keto

One of the best options for beginners of the Ketogenic Diet is going to be cardio! Cardio is great for all ages because you don't have to exercise at high-intensities to gain results. As long as you are getting that heart rate up, you will be able to improve your health in a number of different ways.

When you are doing your cardio, you will want to try your best to maintain a moderate intensity. For this, your target heart rate should be 50-80% of your maximum heart rate. For an average 50-year old, your heart rate should be anywhere between 85 and 119 bpm.

Some of my favorite cardio exercises include:

- Aerobics
- Recreational Sports (with Rest Time)

- Light Circuit Training
- Walking
- Cycling

Tips and Tricks for Maximizing Benefits

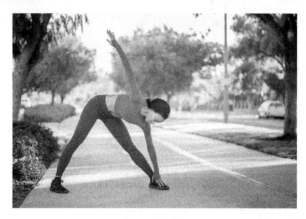

If you do plan on exercising on your diet, the good news is that there are plenty of supplements to help you get to your results quicker and more efficiently. As you pick out your supplements, be sure that they are no-carb. Below, you will find some of my favorite workout supplements.

Creatine
If you are still considering weightlifting on your new diet, you will definitely want to look into purchasing a creatine supplement. This is safe and can enhance your phosphagen system. Generally, you will want to take about five grams a

day to help you increase your power, strength, and muscle mass.

Caffeine

Caffeine is very popular among those who exercise on a regular basis. While it can improve exercise performance, it could potentially decrease your ketone production. For this reason, you will want to consider limiting your caffeine intake, but it works when you really need something at the moment.

MCT Oil

As you learned earlier, MCT is a saturated fat that is digested right away. When you need a boost of energy for endurance or cardio, you can always add some MCT oil to your meal before you exercise. Generally, anywhere between one to two tablespoons should do the trick!

Intermittent Fasting

The last trick I have for you before we dive into the recipes is going to be intermittent fasting! You already know what to eat and how to exercise for the most benefit on your new diet, but Intermittent Fasting will help you get max results from the Ketogenic Diet.

Intermittent fasting is a way of eating that helps you cycle between fasting and eating. While many people feel this is a good way to starve yourself, it is actually a way to help you learn self-control when it comes to eating.

We live in a time where food is easily available. We have grocery stores in every town, McDonald's sprinkled everywhere, and a mass majority of people base their day around meals! As you learn to fast, you will be choosing not to eat anywhere between 12-14 hours.

The basic science behind intermittent fasting is to allow your body to use stored energy. When this happens, it will help you burn excess body fat. When we eat, insulin rises and is stored either in the liver or in the muscle. When it comes to carbohydrates, there is very limited storage space, which is where body fat comes from.

If you are interested in Intermittent Fasting, there are several ways to start. Luckily, you can fast for as short or as long as you would like. What is important is that it fits your schedule, and you see benefits from the actions.

Types of Fasting

- **16/8 Method**
  This first method is one of the more popular versions of Intermittent Fasting. This one allows an 8-10 hour "eating window" with 14-16 hours of fasting. For the 8-10 hours, you can enjoy two or three meals.
- **5:2 Method**

Next, we have the 5:2 method. For this version of Intermittent Fasting, you will normally eat for five days of the week, but for the other two, you will only eat about 500-600 calories in the day.

- **Eat-Stop-Eat**
  Another popular method you could try is the Eat-Stop-Eat. This method of intermittent fasting incorporates 24-hour fasts for either one or two times a week. Of course, I highly suggest starting with the other two before trying this one, but it may work best for your schedule at some point!

Now that you understand the basic concepts of the Ketogenic Diet, we can finally get to the good part, eating! In the next few chapters, you will find some of my top favorite recipes. Each recipe is going to be highly nutritious and will help balance your micro and macronutrients on your new diet. Whether you are looking for a healthy breakfast or a quick snack, you will find a recipe for just about any meal!

Chapter 5: Keto Recipes for Breakfast

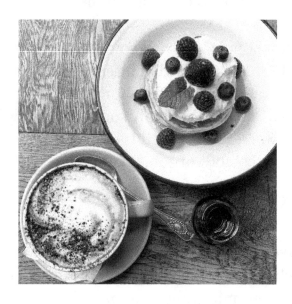

There is nothing quite like starting your morning out with a nice breakfast. The morning is also a great time to get your first boost of fat into your diet and get a boost of energy. Below, you will find some of my favorite, each packed with flavor and nutrition for the Ketogenic Diet.

Spicy Egg Poppers

Yield: Twelve
Time: Forty Minutes

Ingredients

Eggs [8]
Cheddar Cheese [1 C.]
Bacon [10 Strips]
Jalapeno Peppers [4, Diced]
Cream Cheese [3 Ounces]
Salt [Dash]
Garlic Powder [1 t.]
Pepper [Dash]

Directions

1. Egg cups are great to have on hand because they are easy to make and easy to grab if you are short on time! To start this recipe, you will first want to prep your stove to 375.
2. Next, you are going to want to take out a cooking pan and place it over a moderate temperature. Once warm, you will cook the bacon for several minutes. You want to make sure that it isn't cooked through so that you can still bend it a bit. When you are finished, save the bacon grease and place it to the side.
3. When you are ready, you will want to take out a bowl and mend the bacon grease with the eggs, cream cheese, and your seasonings. Once this step is complete, set the bowl aside.

4. Now, it is time to assemble the egg cups. The first step of this process is going to be greasing down a muffin tin and carefully line the walls with your bacon. When the bacon is in place, pour in the egg mixture and be sure that you don't overfill it.
5. The final step is going to be sprinkling the cheese over the top of the egg and then gently placing a jalapeno ring on top. When this is complete, pop the dish into the oven for twenty-five minutes and wait.
6. At the end of this time, the egg should look fluffy and slightly browned at the top. If it is cooked to your liking, remove and enjoy your breakfast!

Macros
- Fats: 25g
- Carbs: 2g
- Proteins: 10g

Stuffed Breakfast Pepper

Yield: Four
Time: Forty Minutes

Ingredients

Bell Pepper [1]
Spinach [1 C.]
Onion [.50, Chopped]
Eggs [2]
Egg Whites [2]
Salsa [Optional]
Pepper [Dash]

Directions

1. These bell peppers are stuffed with flavor and could earn you brownie points for presentation! To start this amazing recipe off, you will first want to prep your stove to 375.
2. As that warms up, take a frying pan and place it over a moderate temperature. When it is warm enough, toss in some olive oil and begin sautéing your onion pieces. If you would like, you can also add in the spinach and salsa for an additional five minutes. When these are cooked to your liking, set them to the side.
3. Next, it is time to get out your baking sheet and line it with tin foil. Once this is complete, carefully slice your bell pepper in half and place the spinach mixture inside of the pepper. With the vegetables placed, you

will then want to carefully spoon in your eggs over the top and then dash some pepper over it.
4. Once the pepper is stuffed, you are going to pop the dish into the oven for half an hour or so. By the end, your eggs should be cooked through and will look fluffy. If they are cooked to your liking, take the dish from the oven and allow them to chill slightly before enjoying.

Macros
- Fats: 5g
- Carbs: 2g
- Proteins: 5g

Keto Breakfast Cookies

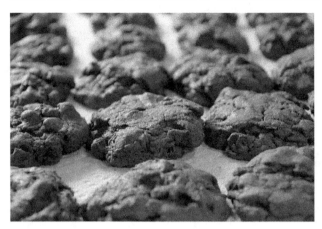

Yield: Twelve
Time: Twenty Minutes

Ingredients

Green Pepper [1, Chopped]
Onion [.50, Chopped]
Sausage [5 Oz.]
Baking Powder [1 t.]
Almond Flour [1 C.]
Eggs [3]
Shredded Cheddar Cheese [1 C.]
Salt [Dash]

Directions
1. Who wouldn't love to have cookies for breakfast? These breakfast "cookies" offer an excellent boost of fats and proteins to your breakfast while keeping your

carb count low. You will want to prepare for this recipe by starting your stove to 375.
2. As this warms up, you can take out your grilling pan and place it over a moderate temperature. Once the pan is heated, add in the peppers, sausage, and the onion and cook for about five or six minutes. By the end, the vegetables should be soft.
3. When these are prepared, get out a sperate bowl and begin beating the eggs with half of the cheese and the flour, baking powder, and the seasoning. Once the sausage and vegetables have cooled enough, you can also add these in.
4. Now that you are all set to stand line tit without can get out a cooking sheet and line it with a silicone mat or paper. Once this is in place, take your dough and place spoonfuls on the surface. When you are ready, add the rest of the cheese over the top and pop into the oven for ten minutes.
5. At the end of this time, your cookies should be golden and can be removed from the oven. Enjoy your breakfast cookie!

Macros
- Fats: 12g
- Carbs: 3g
- Proteins: 10g

Cream Cheese Breakfast Bombs

Yield: Eight
Time: Thirty Minutes

Ingredients

Cream Cheese [1 Package]
Hard-Boiled Eggs [4]
Bacon [1 Pound]
Green Onion [2 T.]

Directions

1. Now that you are starting the Ketogenic Diet, I invite you to the incredible world of fat bombs! Fat bombs are incredible to have on hand, whether you want them for breakfast, a quick snack, or even dessert! This recipe is packed with fat and protein to give you that boost of energy you need in the early morning.
2. To begin this recipe, you will want to boil a pot of water so that you can hard boil your eggs. You can finish this task the way you normally would. Once they are cooked through, you can take the shell off and place it to the side to cool a bit.
3. Next, you will want to get out your frying pan and cook your bacon over a moderate temperature until it is nice and crispy. You will want to follow the directions provided on the side of the package to cook the bacon to your liking. When this step is complete, set the bacon to the side to chill as well.

4. When you are set to make your fat bombs, go ahead and crumble your bacon and chop the hard-boiled egg up into small pieces. Once these items are set, get out the mixing bowl and begin mending the onion, cream cheese, and egg. Once you have your dough, use your hands to roll about eight balls out and place them in the freezer. This will give the balls time to set before rolling them.
5. Now that the balls are slightly hard, you will want to lay your crumbled bacon on a plate and begin rolling the balls in the mixture. You may have to press the ball into the bacon to get it to stick, but don't mush the ball down too much.
6. Finally, your fat bombs are set for your enjoyment!

Macros
- Fats: 40g
- Carbs: 2g
- Proteins: 15g

Cheesy Chive Omelet

Yield: Two
Time: Thirty Minutes

Ingredients

Eggs [4]
Cheddar Cheese [1 C.]
Salt [Dash]
Butter [1 T.]
Chives [1 T.]
Water [.25 C.]
Pepper [Dash]

Directions

1. As you can tell, eggs are extremely popular on the Ketogenic Diet. They are an excellent source of fat and protein to help out with your macros. Adding cheese in the mix is just the frosting on the cake! When you are ready to make this for breakfast, you will want to take out a frying pan and place it over a moderate temperature. It is important to make sure the surface is hot before doing anything.
2. When the pan is heating up, you will want to combine the water, eggs, and seasoning. Once this is set, carefully pour the mixture into your hot pan and wait several minutes. You may need to tilt your pan a bit to create an even omelet.
3. After several minutes, go ahead and sprinkle some of the cheese over half of your omelet. Once in place, you

will want to use a thin spatula to turn half of the omelet over. This takes practice, but if you are gentle enough, you should be able to complete this task with no issue.
4. For a final touch, you are going to go ahead and sprinkle the rest of the cheese over the top of the omelet and continue to cook until it is browned or cooked to your liking.
5. Finally, sprinkle some pepper and salt over the top for some additional flavor, and then your breakfast is set to be served!

Macros
- Fats: 15g
- Carbs: 2g
- Proteins: 8g

Chapter 6: Keto Recipes for Lunch

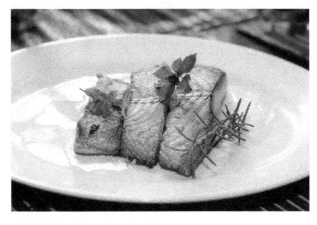

If you are practicing Intermittent Fasting, you will most likely be skipping right to lunch for your first meal. For many people, lunch can be a hard meal to get in because we are at work, at school, or just generally busy. If you plan ahead for lunch, you should have no issues sticking with your diet! Below you will find lunches that are quick and easy to make. Each recipe offers efficient protein and fat to fuel anyone!

Creamy Chicken Salad

Yield: Four
Time: Thirty Minutes

Ingredients

Chicken Breast [1 Lb.]
Avocado [2]
Garlic Cloves [2, Minced]
Lime Juice [3 T.]
Onion [.33 C., Minced]
Jalapeno Pepper [1, Minced]
Salt [Dash]
Cilantro [1 T.]
Pepper [Dash]

Directions
1. If you like traditional chicken salad, this is an excellent alternative to help provide healthier fats along with a good chunk of protein. You will want to start this recipe off my prepping the stove to 400. As this warms up, get out your cooking sheet and line it with paper or foil.
2. Next, it is time to get out the chicken. Go ahead and layer the chicken breast up with some olive oil before seasoning to your liking. I generally use salt and pepper, but feel free to use anything like garlic or onion powder!
3. When the chicken is all set, you will want to line them along the surface of your cooking sheet and pop it into the oven for about twenty minutes. By the end of twenty minutes, the chicken should be cooked through and can be taken out of the oven for chilling. Once cool enough to handle, you will want to either dice or shred your chicken, dependent upon how you like your chicken salad.

4. Now that your chicken is all cooked, it is time to assemble your salad! You can begin this process by adding everything into a bowl and mashing down the avocado. Once your ingredients are mended to your liking, sprinkle some salt over the top and serve immediately. Whether you like your chicken salad straight out of the bowl or in a low-carb wrap, it can be enjoyed in a number of different ways!

Macros
- Fats: 20g
- Carbs: 4g
- Proteins: 25g

Spicy Keto Chicken Wings

Yield: Four
Time: One Hour

Ingredients

Chicken Wings [2 Lbs.]
Cajun Spice [1 t.]
Smoked Paprika [2 t.]
Turmeric [.50 t.]
Salt [Dash]
Baking Powder [2 t.]
Pepper [Dash]

Directions

1. When you first begin the Ketogenic Diet, you may find that you won't be eating the traditional foods that may have made up a majority of your diet in the past. While this is a good thing for your health, you may feel you are missing out! The good news is that there are delicious alternatives that aren't lacking in flavor! To start this recipe, you'll want to prep the stove to 400.
2. As this heats up, you will want to take some time to dry your chicken wings with a paper towel. This will help remove any excess moisture and get you some nice, crispy wings!
3. When you are all set, take out a mixing bowl and place all of the seasonings along with the baking powder. If you feel like it, you can adjust the seasoning levels

however you would like. Once these are set, go ahead and throw the chicken wings in and coat evenly. If you have one, you'll want to place the wings on a wire rack that is placed over your baking tray. If not, you can just lay them across the baking sheet.
4. Now that your chicken wings are set, you are going to pop them into the stove for thirty minutes. By the end of this time, the tops of the wings should be crispy. If they are, take them out from the oven and flip them so that you can bake the other side. You will want to cook these for an additional thirty minutes.
5. Finally, take the tray from the oven and allow to cool slightly before serving up your spiced keto wings. For additional flavor, serve with any of your favorite, keto-friendly dipping sauce.

Macros
- Fats: 7g
- Carbs: 1g
- Proteins: 60g

Cilantro and Lime Creamed Chicken

Yield: Four
Time: Thirty Minutes

Ingredients

Chicken Breast [4 Pieces]
Red Pepper Flakes [1 t.]
Cilantro [1 T.]
Salt [Dash]
Lime Juice [2 T.]
Chicken Broth [1 C.]
Onion [.25 C., Chopped]
Olive Oil [1 T.]
Heavy Cream [.50 C.]
Pepper [Dash]

Directions

1. If you are looking for a dish that is a bit different, this recipe is going to be perfect for you. Between the cilantro and the lime, this dish offers a fresh twist on traditional chicken. Many people feel that in order to lose weight, they need to give up flavor, but on the Ketogenic Diet, that is simply not the case! To begin this recipe, you will want to get out your cooking skillet and place it over a moderate temperature.
2. As the skillet heats, go ahead and season the chicken breast according to your taste. For this particular

recipe, you will want to consider using the seasonings provided in the list above, but feel free to adjust levels to your own taste. Once seasoned to your liking, throw the chicken into the skillet and cook for about eight minutes on each side. When the chicken is cooked through, take it out of the pan and place to the side.
3. Next, you are going to add the onion into the hot pan and cook them for a minute before also adding in the cilantro, pepper flakes, lime juice, and the chicken broth. If you don't have chicken broth on hand, feel free to use water. Once these items are in place, bring to a boil for ten minutes.
4. Last-minute, you are going to whisk in your heavy cream and add in the chicken so that it can be coated in the sauce you just made. For extra flavor, add in some more cilantro, and then your chicken can be served by itself or with a keto-friendly vegetable!

Macros
- Fats: 20g
- Carbs: 6g
- Proteins: 30g

Cheesy Ham Quiche

Yield: Six
Time: Forty Minutes

Ingredients

Eggs [8]
Zucchini [1 C., Shredded]
Heavy Cream [.50 C.]
Ham [1 C., Diced]
Mustard [1 t.]
Salt [Dash]

Directions

1. Unlike traditional quiche, this version is crustless! Because there is no crust, this recipe offers a low-carb option for those who are still looking to make a savory meal for breakfast or lunch. For this recipe, you can start off by prepping your stove to 375 and getting out a pie plate for your quiche.
2. Next, it is time to prep the zucchini. First, you will want to go ahead and shred it into small pieces. Once this is complete, take a paper towel and gently squeeze out the excess moisture. This will help avoid a soggy quiche.
3. When the step from above is complete, you will want to place the zucchini into your pie plate along with the cooked ham pieces and your cheese. Once these items are in place, you will want to whisk the seasonings,

cream, and eggs together before pouring it over the top.
4. Now that your quiche is set, you are going to pop the dish into your stove for about forty minutes. By the end of this time, the egg should be cooked through, and you will be able to insert a knife into the center and have it come out clean.
5. If the quiche is cooked to your liking, take the dish from the oven and allow it to chill slightly before slicing and serving.

Macros
- Fats: 25g
- Carbs: 2g
- Proteins: 20g

Loaded Cauliflower Rice

Yield: Four
Time: Thirty Minutes

Ingredients
Cauliflower [1 Head]
Cheddar Cheese [1 C.]
Bacon [1 Lb.]
Chives [.50 C.]
Salt [Dash]

Directions
1. Sometimes, you just want something basic for lunch. This loaded cauliflower rice is fairly easy to make and only requires a handful of ingredients! The first step of this recipe is going to be ricing your cauliflower. You can choose to do this by hand, or you can purchase cauliflower rice in the frozen section.
2. Next, you will want to take several moments to cook your bacon. You can complete this task by heating a grilling pan over a moderate temperature and cook the bacon for four or five minutes on either side. I like my bacon crispy, but that is completely up to you!
3. When you are set, you are going to place your cauliflower rice into a microwave-safe bowl and sprinkle your shredded cheese over the top. When this is set, go ahead and pop the bowl into the microwave for a minute and allow for the rice to cook through and the cheese to melt.

4. Once the step from above is complete, top the dish off with your bacon pieces and season to your liking. Just like that, lunch will be ready for you!

Macros
- Fats: 10g
- Carbs: 5g
- Proteins: 5g

Chapter 7: Keto Recipes for Dinner

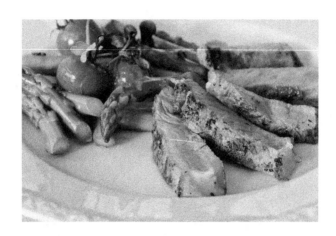

Dinner is a very important meal for the day. Whether you are cooking for one or cooking for your whole family, dinner can truly bring people together. Hopefully, at this point in your day, you will be able to take some time to slow down and enjoy the process of cooking. If not, there are plenty of recipes that are still quick and easy to make — the recipes to follow range for a variety of flavors for just about anyone.

Buttery Garlic Steak

Yield: Four
Time: Thirty Minutes

Ingredients
Steak [1 Lb.]

Grass-fed Butter [5 T.]
Garlic Cloves [5 T., Minced]
Parsley [.25 C.]
Salt [Dash]

Directions
1. One of the secret tips I can give you for the Ketogenic Diet is to put butter on absolutely everything that you can. Vegetable? Butter. Side dish? Butter. Main dish? Butter! This garlic butter steak is out of this world and incredibly easy to make. Before you even think about cooking, you will want to set aside several moments to season your steak properly. The best technique to use would be patting the steak down and then season with pepper and salt on both sides. Be generous with your seasoning!
2. Next, it is time to cook your steak. If you have a heavy-duty skillet, use it! Once you have your skillet, bring it over a moderate temperature and heat for several minutes without anything in it. Once hot, add in the steak and sear both sides for about three minutes. If you like your steak cooked past medium-rare, leave it on longer. When the steak is cooked to your liking, remove it from the pan and set to the side.
3. Now that your steak is cooked through, it is time to make the garlic butter. To accomplish this, you will want to lower the heat in your skillet and begin melting your butter. Once the butter has been liquified, you will next add in the garlic and cook for

an additional minute. When the garlic turns a golden color, take the pan away from the heat.
4. The next step will be slicing up your steak. Once it is complete, carefully drizzle your butter sauce over the top until the steak becomes completely coated. As a final touch, garnish with some fresh parsley and enjoy your dinner.

Macros
- Fats: 25g
- Carbs: 2g
- Proteins: 25g

Baked Lemon Salmon

Yield: Four
Time: Twenty Minutes

Ingredients
Salmon [4 Pieces]
Salt [Dash]
Lemon Juice [2 T.]
Lemon [1]
Grass-fed Butter [2 T.]
Pepper [Dash]

Directions
1. If you enjoy your fresh seafood, this lemon salmon fillet is going to blow your mind. The lemon offers a refreshing twist to the fish and goes perfect with a side of cauliflower or broccoli. To start this recipe off, you will first want to go ahead and prep the stove to 400. As it heats up, get out your baking sheet and line it.
2. When you are set to cook the fish, you will first want to run it under water before patting it down with some paper towels. Once this has been done, place the fish with the skin side facing down.
3. Next, you will melt your butter and carefully spoon it over each piece of fish. With the butter in place, you can season with some pepper and salt according to your own taste.

4. Now that the fish has been seasoned, you will then want to pour your lemon juice over the top and place a slice of lemon on top of each salmon filet.
5. When you are ready to cook your meal, you are now going to pop the dish into the stove for fifteen minutes. By the end of this time, you will know that your fish is cooked through if you can flake it easily with a fork. If it is cooked through, take the dish out from the oven and allow it to chill for several minutes.
6. Finally, serve the fish with your favorite keto-friendly side, and enjoy your meal.

Macros
- Fats: 20g
- Carbs: 3g
- Proteins: 20g

One Sheet Fajitas

Yield: Six
Time: Twenty Minutes

Ingredients

Chicken Breast [1 Lb.]
Fajita Seasoning [2 T.]
Cilantro [.25 C.]
Onion [1, Sliced]
Red Bell Pepper [1, Sliced]
Green Bell Pepper [1, Sliced]
Olive Oil [3 T.]
Salt [Dash]
Lime Juice [2 T.]

Directions

1. What is better than fajitas for dinner? Fajitas that you can make using one pan! This recipe is easy to make and easy to enjoy. To begin, you will want to go ahead and prep the oven to 400. As this warms up, you can also get out the one baking sheet it is going to take for this recipe.
2. When you are all set, you will want to throw all of the ingredients from above into a mixing bowl and season with the pepper, salt, and the lime juice. Once this is set, spread the items across your baking sheet as evenly as possible.
3. Now that your sheet is set, you are going to pop it into the stove for twenty minutes. By the end of this time,

the chicken should be cooked through. If you like everything a little crispy, you can go ahead and broil the ingredients for an additional two minutes.
4. When your meal is set, take it out from the stove and allow it to chill for two minutes. As a final touch, season with some fresh cilantro and enjoy your keto-friendly fajitas!

Macros
- Fats: 10g
- Carbs: 4g
- Proteins: 25g

Balsamic Chicken

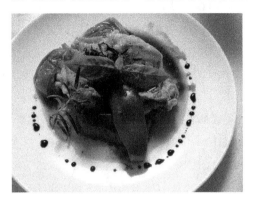

Yield: Four
Time: One Hour

Ingredients

Chicken Breast [4 Pieces]
Grass-fed Butter [2 T.]
Salt [Dash]
Roasted Garlic Cloves [4]
Mushrooms [2 C., Sliced]
Thyme [1 t.]
Chives [1 T.]
Red Pepper Flakes [1 t.]
Balsamic Vinegar [.25 C.]
Water [.50 C.]
Onions [.25 C., Chopped]

Directions

1. While following the Ketogenic Diet, it is a good idea to always have chicken on hand. This is a very versatile

item and can offer a pack of protein as long as it is paired with the proper fats to balance out your diet. While this recipe does take a bit longer, the flavor will be worth the wait. You can begin this recipe by prepping the stove to 350 and getting out your baking sheet.

2. As the stove warms up, you will want to take out your skillet and begin heating the butter in it. Once the butter is melted, add in the chicken pieces and season with your pepper and salt. When the meat is seasoned to your liking, grill each side of the chicken for three or four minutes. Once the chicken is cooked through, place it onto your baking sheet, and cook in your heated stove for an additional twenty-five minutes.

3. As the chicken cooks, you will want to melt some more butter in your heated pan. Once melted, add in your mushrooms and onions. You will want to sauté these items for a minute before adding in the roasted garlic, thyme, red pepper flakes, and the balsamic vinegar. After these ingredients have cooked for a minute, pour in the water and stir until the liquid begins to reduce.

4. Finally, you are going to pour the mixture over your chicken and serve the dish hot. If you would like, you can serve with fresh parsley or chopped chives for some nice additional flavors.

Macros
- Fats: 15g
- Carbs: 8g

➢ Proteins: 30g

Cheesy Keto Meatballs

Yield: Three
Time: Twenty Minutes

Ingredients

Ground Beef [1 Lb.]
Salt [Dash]
Garlic Powder [1 t.]
Parmesan Cheese [3 T.]
Mozzarella Cheese [1 C.]
Pepper [Dash]

Directions
1. Whether you are looking for a snack to pop into your mouth quickly or a delicious meal, this recipe can help you out. While meatballs are delicious by themselves, imagine stuffing them with cheese. To begin this recipe, you will want to take some time to chop your fresh mozzarella into bite-sized pieces.
2. When this first step is complete, season the ground beef to your liking and then carefully wrap each cheese piece with the ground beef and begin creating your meatballs. This recipe should make between nine and ten balls.
3. Once you are set to cook your meal, you will want to take out your frying pan and place it over a moderate temperature. When the pan is warm, you can go

ahead and grill the meatballs on all sides for five minutes or so. By the end of this time, the meatballs should be crispy and can be served over some zoodles or enjoyed by themselves!

Macros
- Fats: 35g
- Carbs: 2g
- Proteins: 40g

Chapter 8: Keto Salad Recipes

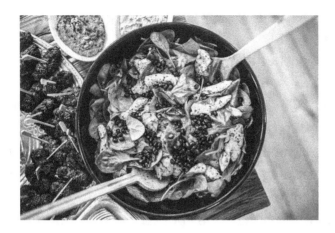

For a quick and easy meal, it is a great idea to have salads on hand. These can be staples in your diet, whether you are eating salad for lunch or dinner. If you incorporate any of these meals throughout the week, it can help you save time and stick to your diet on the busiest of days.

Pesto Chicken Salad

Yield: Four
Time: Thirty Minutes

Ingredients

Chicken Breast [4 Pieces]
Pesto [.50 C.]
Cherry Tomatoes [1 C.]
Spinach [3 C.]

Salt [Dash]
Olive Oil [3 T.]

Directions
1. For another alternative for plain old, baked chicken, you will want to consider this delicious Pesto chicken salad! To start off, you are going to want to go ahead and prep the stove to 350. As this warms up, place your chicken pieces onto a baking plate and coat with the pepper, salt, and olive oil. When this is done, pop the dish into the oven for forty minutes.
2. When the chicken is cooked through and no longer pink on the inside, you will now take it away from the oven and cool slightly before handling.
3. Once you can handle the chick, you will want to toss it into a bowl along with the pesto and your sliced tomatoes. When the ingredients are mended to your liking, place over a bowl of fresh spinach and enjoy your salad.

Macros
- Fats: 12g
- Carbs: 2g
- Proteins: 40g

Fresh Summer Salad

Yield: Four
Time: Ten Minutes

Ingredients

Olive Oil [2 T.]
Thyme [1 t.]
Oregano [1 t.]
Ricotta Cheese [.25 C.]
Basil [1 Leaf, Chopped]
Balsamic Vinegar [1 T.]
Cucumber [1, Sliced]
Tomato [3, Sliced]
Radishes [5, Sliced]
Onion [1, Sliced]

Directions

1. Don't be fooled by the name; this salad can be enjoyed at any time of the year! If you are looking for a meatless dish, this is the perfect recipe for you! The first step you will want to take for this recipe will be making your ricotta cheese. You can complete this in a small bowl by mending the thyme, oregano, basil in with the ricotta cheese.
2. Next, you will be making your own dressing! For this task, all you have to do is whisk your vinegar and olive oil together. Once this is complete, season however you would like.

3. Finally, take some time to slice and dice the vegetables according to the directions above. When your veggies are all set, you will want to assemble them in your serving dishes and pour the dressing generously over the top. As a final touch, dollop your ricotta cheese over your salad, and then your salad will be ready for serving.

Macros
- Fats: 10g
- Carbs: 8g
- Proteins: 5g

Keto Taco Salad

Yield: Six
Time: Twenty Minutes

Ingredients

Ground Beef [1 Ln.]
Olive Oil [3 T.]
Pepper [Dash]
Onion Powder [1 T.]
Cumin [1 T.]
Garlic Clove [1 T., Minced]
Tomato [1, Chopped]
Sour Cream [.50 C.]
Black Olives [.50 C.]
Cheddar Cheese [.25 C.]
Cilantro [2 T.]
Green Pepper [1, Chopped]

Directions

1. With taco salad, you will be able to enjoy everything that you love about tacos with a lot less carbohydrates! Whether you prepare this for taco Tuesday or a quick lunch, it is sure to be a crowd-pleaser!
2. Start this recipe off by taking out your grilling pan and place it over a moderate temperature. As it warms up, you can add in the olive oil and let that sizzle. When you are set, add in the green pepper, spices, and ground beef. You can also use ground turkey in

this recipe if that is more your style. Go ahead and cook these ingredients together for ten minutes or so.
3. When you are all set, place some mixed greens into a bowl and cover with the meat mixture you just created. If you would like some extra flavor, sprinkle some cheddar cheese over the top along with some sour cream.

Macros
- Fats: 20g
- Carbs: 5g
- Proteins: 20g

Mixed Vegetable Tuna Salad

Yield: Four
Time: Ten Minutes

Ingredients

Canned Tuna [1 Can]
Olive Oil [2 T.]
Parsley [.25 C.]
Red Pepper [1, Roasted & Chopped]
Artichoke Hearts [.50 C., Diced]
Black Olives [.25 C.]
Basil [2 T.]
Lemon Juice [2 T.}
Pepper [Dash]

Directions

1. When you are in a rush, you can't go wrong with tuna salad! To save yourself even more time, you can go ahead and prep this tuna salad at the beginning of the week so that all you will have to do is grab and go!
2. For this recipe, get out a mixing bowl and mend all of the items from the list above. Once combined, feel free to season with pepper and salt to your liking.
3. For serving purposes, this tuna salad can be enjoyed in a number of different ways. You can eat it right out of the bowl, scooped into a lettuce wrap, or served over a bed of salad!

Macros

- Fats: 15g
- Carbs: 3g
- Proteins: 10g

Lemon Shrimp Salad

Yield: Four
Time: Twenty Minutes

Ingredients

Mixed Greens [5 C.]
Olive Oil [2 T.]
Shrimp [1 Lb.]
Sliced Almonds [.25 C.]
Avocado [2, Sliced]
Pepper [Dash]
Lemon Juice [2 T.]

Directions

1. When people think about making a salad for lunch, they often think of either chicken or steak over the top. Have you ever considered shrimp on your salad? It is an awesome alternative when you don't feel like having chicken or steak again. To begin this recipe, you will first need to sear your shrimp.
2. For some added flavor, go ahead and mix your shrimp with some pepper and lemon juice. When it is coated to your liking, you are going to place it into a grilling pan over a moderate temperature. We are only going

to sear the shrimp so it should only take two to three minutes on either side. You will just want to make sure that the shrimp is cooked thoroughly.
3. When the shrimp is cooked to your liking, it is time to assemble your salad. Go ahead and place your mixed greens into your serving bowls and squeeze some lemon juice over the top. Once these items are in place, add in the olive oil and begin layering the avocado on top.
4. For a final touch, add in the shrimp and sliced almonds for a bit of a crunch. Just like that, your salad will be fresh and ready for serving.

Macros
- Fats: 30g
- Carbs: 10g
- Proteins: 30g

Chapter 9: Keto Recipes for Snacks

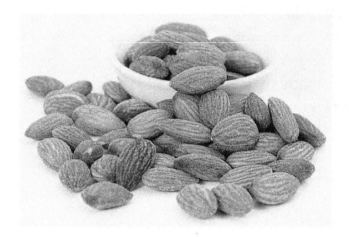

As you begin the Ketogenic Diet, you may find it surprising, but many people find that their meals are filling enough that they don't need a snack in the first place! However, if you are going to snack, you will want to make sure that it is Keto-friendly.

In this chapter, you will find some quick and easy keto snacks to help you get started. Keep in mind that if you are looking to lose weight on your new diet, you will need to keep your calories and snacking to a minimum. You may find that you are hungry to begin with, but it will get better with time!

Sweet Cinnamon Roll Fat Bomb

Yield: Twenty
Time: Ten Minutes

Ingredients

Cream Cheese [1 Package]
Stevia [.25 C.]
Grass-fed Butter [.50 C.]
Heavy Whipping Cream [3 T.]
Vanilla Extract [.25 t.]
Stevia [2 T.]
Ground Cinnamon {2 t.}
Almond Flour [1 C.]
Cream Cheese [1 Oz.]

Directions
1. When you are first starting the Ketogenic Diet, it is a good idea to always have fat bombs on hand. If you are experiencing symptoms from the Keto-Flu or are just feeling a little tired, a fat bomb should be able to pick you right up!
2. You will begin this recipe by making the balls. In order to do this, you will want to soften your first package of cream cheese and mend it in a bowl with your softened butter. Once these are combined well, you can add in the vanilla extract.
3. Next, you will add in your ground cinnamon and flour. Now that you have your dough, you will want to use your hands to create balls. Generally, you should

be able to make anywhere between fifteen and twenty fat bombs. When this step is complete, pop the dish into your freezer for thirty minutes so that they can set.
4. Your next step is going to be making your frosting. You can complete this task by combining the vanilla extract with your heavy whipping cream, cream cheese, and a touch of sweetener.
5. When your balls are solid enough, remove from the freezer and place onto your counter. Here, you can begin to drizzle or dunk the balls into your frosting and then put back into the freezer.
6. After an additional ten minutes or so, your snack will be set for your enjoyment!

Macros
- Fats: 15g
- Carbs: 1g
- Proteins: 2g

Sausage and Cheese Puffs

Yield: Four
Time: Thirty Minutes

Ingredients

Butter [4 T., Melted]
Cheddar Cheese [2 C.]
Sausage [1 Lb.]
Eggs [4}
Garlic Powder [.25 t.]
Baking Powder [.25 t.]
Coconut Flour [.25 C.]
Sour Cream [3 T.]
Salt [Dash]

Directions

1. For another quick and easy snack, you will want to try these little balls of heaven! They are soft, fluffy, and offer a good chunk of fat when you need it! This recipe can be used as a snack or can be an excellent addition to breakfast as well! To start off, you will want to prep the stove to 375. You can also get out a baking sheet; you are going to need it later.
2. Next, it is time to get out the griddle! Go ahead and bring it over a moderate temperature. As it warms up, place your butter and let it melt. Once it is melted, add in your sausage and cook on both sides. Generally, this should only take three or four minutes.

When it is cooked to your liking, take it out from the pan and set to the side.
3. Your next step will require a mixing bowl. Once you have your bowl, mend together the garlic, salt, sour cream, eggs, and four tablespoons of melted butter. When these are combined, add in the baking powder and coconut flour. Now that your dough is created, you will also want to fold in the cooked sausage and your shredded cheese.
4. Next, you will want to take your hands and make balls of batter. As you do this, line them up evenly across the surface of your baking sheet. When this is set, pop the dish into the stove for twenty minutes. By the end, the balls should be browned and cooked through.
5. If they are cooked to your liking, take the dish from the stove and chill slightly before digging into your snack.

Macros
- Fats: 50g
- Carbs: 2g
- Proteins: 30g

Frozen Berry Bites

Yield: Four
Time: Three Hours

Ingredients

Milk [2 T.]
Full-fat Yogurt [2 C.]
Blackberries [.25 C.]
Raspberries [.25 C.]
Stevia [1 Packet]

Directions

1. As you learned in the second chapter, fruit is generally left out of the Ketogenic Diet because it is high in sugar and carbs. However, sometimes it is nice to have as a treat! You will note that this recipe is slightly higher in carbohydrates, but as long as you count it with your macros, you can still enjoy some frozen berry bites in moderation!
2. To begin this recipe, you will first want to take some time to mash down the fruit into smaller pieces. When this is complete, you can add in your milk and yogurt. Once in place, combine everything together as well as possible so that the fruit is spread evenly.
3. When you are set, pour the mixture into an ice cube tray and pop into the freezer for about three hours. By the end, you can pop out the chunks, and your berry bites will be set for snack time.

Macros
- Fats: 5g
- Carbs: 7g
- Proteins: 5g

Cream Cheese and Ham Rolls

Yield: Four
Time: Five Minutes

Ingredients

Dill Pickles [15]
Cream Cheese [1 Package]
Sliced Ham [15 Slices]

Directions

1. When you need a quick snack, this is the perfect recipe to whip together. Plus, finger foods can be a lot of fun if you are trying to get a child or friend to try out the Ketogenic Diet!
2. To make this quick and easy snack, you will first want to lay out each slice of ham in front of you. When this is done, carefully spread about a tablespoon of cream cheese across the surface. You will want to do this carefully because the ham can tear easily if the slices are not thick enough.
3. Finally, you are going to place one small pickle into the center and roll it up tightly. If needed, you can use a toothpick to keep your rolls in place.

4. When the step from above is complete, pop the dish into the fridge for at least two hours before serving.

Macros
- Fats: 30g
- Carbs: 6g
- Proteins: 20g

Keto-friendly Crackers

Yield: Twenty-five
Time: Twenty Minutes

Ingredients

Almond Flour [2 C.]
Eggs [2]
Grass-fed Butter [8 T., Soft]
Salt [Dash]

Directions

1. While these crackers don't particularly offer a high amount of fat or protein, this recipe is great to have on hand. Crackers are versatile, whether you are looking for a snack or something on the side. You will find that many crackers in the market are filled with additives and high in carbs. To help keep them keto-friendly, you can make your own! To start out, prep the stove to 350 and get out your favorite baking sheet.

2. When you are set, take out a bowl and mend together the almond flour with the softened butter. For this step, it can be extremely helpful to have a hand mixer!
3. Once these two items are blended together, add in your eggs one at a time and punch some salt over the top. You will want to continue stirring these items until you get a perfectly smooth dough.
4. Next, you will want to place the dough in between two pieces of parchment paper and begin rolling out the dough onto your baking sheet. By doing this, you can make sure that the dough is flat and even. You will want to roll the dough out until it is about an eighth of an inch in thickness.
5. When you are done rolling the dough, use a pizza cutter to score your dough. You can make the crackers as big or as small as you would like! Once you have cut the dough up, pop the dish into the stove for fifteen minutes. By the end, the crackers should be golden.
6. As a final touch, sprinkle some more salt over the top, and then your crackers will be all ready for you to enjoy!

Macros
- Fats: 10g
- Carbs: 1g
- Proteins: 2g

Chapter 10: Keto Recipes for Dessert

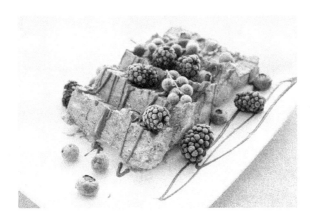

Last but not least, we will end this book on the sweetest part of the day, dessert! While other diets normally discourage anything sweet or along the lines of dessert, you will be able to enjoy keto-friendly desserts on your new diet!

Much like with snacking, you will want to consider keeping dessert to a minimum if you are looking to lose weight on your diet. Remember that the only way you are going to lose weight is if you have a calorie deficit. For this reason, I suggest only indulging in dessert once or twice a week. If you have the macros left for it, I say go for it!

Chocolate Peanut Butter Bombs

Yield: Ten
Time: Five Minutes

Ingredients

Almond Flour [2 T.]
Stevia [2 T.]
Vanilla Extract [.25 t.]
Olive Oil [1 T.]
Peanut Butter [.25 C.]
Chocolate Chips [.50 C.]

Directions

1. Is there a better combination than peanut butter and chocolate? When you put these two things together, you will have a delicious and keto-friendly dessert ready when you need it. To start out, you will want to get out your mixing bowl so that you can mend the flour, sweetener, peanut butter, and vanilla extract. From this, you will get your dough.
2. When you are all set, you can use your hands to roll balls from this mixture. With this recipe, you should be able to make between ten and twelve balls. Once these are set, you will want to place them on a plate and pop into the freezer for half an hour.
3. After the balls have set and are on the harder side, remove from the freezer and place back onto the counter. Now, you will want to carefully melt your chocolate chips in a microwave-safe bowl. Generally,

this will only take thirty to forty seconds. Make sure you watch the chocolate chips because they can burn fairly easily.
4. Once the chocolate has been melted, carefully dip each ball into the melted chocolate and coat evenly. If you would like, you can also drizzle the chocolate over the top. Once you have put the chocolate on the balls, you will want to place the plate of balls back into the freezer for an additional fifteen minutes.
5. Once this time has passed, the chocolate peanut butter balls will be ready for dessert! Enjoy!

Macros
- Fats: 5g
- Carbs: 1g
- Proteins: 3g

Keto Ice Cream

Yield: Ten
Time: Thirty Minutes

Ingredients

Egg Yolks [2]
Creamy Peanut Butter [.50 C.]
Heavy Whipping Cream [2 C.]
Cocoa Powder, Unsweetened [2 T.]
Erythritol [.50 C.]

Directions

1. When you first start the Ketogenic Diet, you will quickly learn that all of your favorite foods are going to be high in carbs, high in added sugar, and filled with additives that are bad for your health. Luckily, you will be able to make a majority of your favorites all on your own! Here, we have a simple chocolate and peanut butter ice cream that only requires five ingredients!
2. The first step of making your own ice cream will be taking out a mixing bowl and dissolving your cocoa powder. For this, you will only need about two tablespoons of water. When this is set, place it into a food processor with the rest of the ingredients and mend everything together for a few seconds.
3. When this is set, you are going to pour the mixture into a bowl and freeze for around three hours. After this, you will have delicious ice cream that is still

keto-friendly! If you have an ice cream maker, you can also pour the mixture into here and have ice cream almost in an instant!

Macros
- Fats: 30g
- Carbs: 4g
- Proteins: 5g

Cheesecake Fat Bombs

Yield: Fifteen
Time: Thirty Minutes

Ingredients

Fresh Raspberries [.25 C.]
Cream Cheese [1 Package]
Stevia [2 T.]
Grass-fed Butter [3 T.]
Vanilla Extract [1 T.]

Directions

1. If you are a fan of cheesecake, you are going to absolutely love this recipe. By making these fat bombs, it is a great way to eat your cheesecake guilt-free because it is keto-friendly! Though it is delicious, remember to keep your dessert in moderation! Calories still count as calories, and there is such thing as too much fat on the Ketogenic Diet. You have to find the balance while still enjoying your treats.

2. To start this recipe, you will want to take some time to mash your raspberries down into smaller bits. Once the raspberry has been smashed, add in the cream cheese and the butter. To make this easier, you can leave the cream cheese and butter out at room temperature for around an hour or so.
3. Now that you have your mixture take your hands to create balls from the dough and place it into your freezer for thirty minutes. At the end of this time, your fat bombs will be solid and set for dessert.

Macros
- Fats: 10g
- Carbs: 1g
- Proteins: 2g

Lemon Bars

Yield: Eight
Time: One Hour

Ingredients

Almond Flour [2 C.]
Lemons [2]
Eggs [3]
Erythritol [1 C.]
Butter [.25 C.]

Directions

1. Not everyone is a chocolate lover, and that is okay to admit! These lemon bars are dense and fluffy. If you need something to bring to a party, this is the perfect recipe to try out! You don't have to be following a Ketogenic Diet to enjoy this one.
2. You will want to start this recipe off by prepping the stove to 350. As the stove heats up, line your baking dish with some paper and begin mixing together the almond flour with the erythritol. For a touch more of flavor, feel free to add a pinch of salt.
3. When you are set, pour the mixture into your baking dish and pop it into the stove for twenty minutes. By the end of this time, the bars should be set and can be taken out of the oven.
4. Next, it is time to make the lemon zest for your bars! In a bowl, you will want to juice the two lemons and add the zest from one. When these are set, mix in

your eggs along with a cup of erythritol and another cup of your almond flour. Once this step is complete, pour it onto the crust and pop the dish back into the stove for an additional twenty-five minutes.

5. When your bars are cooked to your liking, take the dish from the oven and allow it to chill for ten minutes before slicing the bars up. For a finishing touch, sprinkle some more erythritol over the top and even decorate with a slice of lemon!

Macros
- Fats: 25g
- Carbs: 5g
- Proteins: 7g

Ketogenic Cookie Dough

Yield: Four
Time: Ten Minutes

Ingredients

Cream Cheese [1 Package]
Dark Chocolate Chips [.25 C.]
Grass-fed Butter [2 T.]
Vanilla Extract [1 T.]
Creamy Peanut Butter [5 T.]
Stevia [.25 C.]

Directions

1. We are all guilty of eating raw cookie dough. Now, you can enjoy raw cookie dough on purpose, while still following your diet! This is another version of a fat bomb, meaning you can enjoy it as a dessert or make other people extremely jealous of your delicious snack!
2. To make these fat bombs, you are going to take all of the ingredients from the list above, minus the chocolate chips, and place them into your food processor. Once you have created your dough, you will next fold in your chocolate chips.
3. When this step is complete, use your hands to create small balls from the dough. As you do this, you will want to place each ball onto a plate so that you can place the plate into the freezer for thirty minutes.
4. After this time has passed, you will have fat bombs for dessert! Enjoy!

Macros

- Fats: 20g
- Carbs: 6g
- Proteins: 5g

Conclusion

Thank you for making it through to the end of *Keto After 50: The Ultimate Guide to Ketogenic Diet for Men and Women Over 50*, let's hope it was informative and able to provide you with all of the tools you need to achieve your goals whatever they may be.

Beginning the Keto diet can seem daunting at first, but you have all of the information you need to help you get started! I hope that you find the courage and motivation to follow your new lifestyle so that you can experience all of the incredible benefits that come with the diet.

If you ever have any questions, feel free to use this book as your ultimate guide. There are going to be bumps along the way, but you are very well prepared at this point. Remember that there is no point in giving up! The Ketogenic Diet works, the science is proof! As long as you follow the rules, keep your carbs to a minimum, and eat the foods you are supposed to, you are going to see the results in no time! All you have to do is put in the work!

Finally, if you found this book useful in any way, a review on Amazon is always appreciated!

Keto for Women Over 50

The Ultimate Guide for Senior Women to Ketogenic Diet and a Healthy Weight Loss, Including Mouthwatering Recipes to Reset Your Metabolism and Boost your Energy

Thomas Slow

Introduction

Congratulations on purchasing *Keto For Women Over 50,* and thank you for doing so.

This book is for women over 50 looking to lose weight and increase energy levels through the ketogenic (keto) diet. Naysayers will say the keto diet is a fad, but some form of this diet has been used for various health purposes, including weight loss, since 1825. Over the last 200 years, the diet has been changed and adjusted to incorporate the newest scientific information into the diet. As a result, the keto diet takes an age-old concept of limiting carbohydrates with the current knowledge of how fats work in the human body and now the diet is better than ever. The weight loss, when adapting the keto diet, is almost immediate. This book provides a basic framework for losing weight and improving your health by adopting a low-carbohydrate, high-fat diet. Your questions will be answered. By now, you've probably realized that it is not as easy to lose weight as it was when you were younger. That is probably the result of a lot of things; a slowing metabolism and decreased mobility are the obvious reasons you may be gaining weight, but the food you eat may be a culprit as well. Reading this book, you will be able to completely restructure your life and diet to follow ketogenic principles. The ketogenic diet is designed to help you lose weight with an increased energy level. This book outlines the basics and has the information to get you started. As a bonus, you will receive over 20 recipes that follow the keto diet principles. These recipes give you an opportunity to find new and creative ways to prepare food when you are starting out and may not be familiar with all the foods on the plan. There is also a food list inside that you can use to plan meals and purchase groceries for your new lighter, healthier lifestyle.

There happens to be a lot of books out there on this subject. Thank you for purchasing this one! I made sure it is jam packed with helpful information to get you where you want to be. Enjoy!

Chapter 1: Keto – An Overview

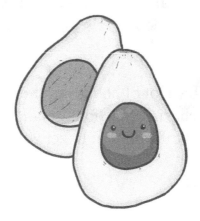

What is the Keto Diet?

Before you start the ketogenic diet, you will want to know what it is. The diet, at its most basic, is the replacement of carbohydrates with fats. This makes the keto diet not only a low carb diet but a very low carb diet. The food consumed on the keto diet will be high in fat with the reduction of carbs. When you limit the number of carbohydrates in your body, you will get your energy from stored fat. This is called ketosis. When your body is in ketosis, it is in a metabolic state that causes it to burn fat for energy instead of carbohydrates. This is the state we strive to reach on the diet; energy from fat.

There are four types of keto diets:

1. The standard ketogenic diet (SKD) is the basic ketogenic diet. This diet allows for 75% of the calories consumed to be from fat, 20% of the calories from protein, and 5% carbohydrates.
2. The cyclical ketogenic diet (CKD) is designed so that the dieter follows the Standard Ketogenic Diet for 5 days each week, followed by 2 days of high carbohydrates. CKD is used for people attempting to increase muscle and strength.
3. The targeted ketogenic diet (TKD) is used by people who need extra energy to get through strenuous workouts or training. The carbohydrates can be consumed either before or after a workout to provide extra energy for the short term.
4. On the high protein ketogenic diet (HPKD) is used for people who do not want to lose muscle mass like bodybuilders and older people. The percentage of protein in the diet can go up to 35% with fat decreasing as low as 60%, with the carbohydrates remaining at 5%.

The ketogenic diet is based on science. When the body does not have carbohydrates to use as energy, fat is used instead. This process is called ketogenesis, and the body generates. During this process, ketones are generated by the liver. The average person can safely get up to 70% of its energy from ketones. It takes about three weeks for the body to transform itself from using carbohydrates for energy to efficiently using ketones for energy.

What is Ketosis?

Ketosis is a metabolic state where the body is efficiently using fat for energy. In a regular diet, carbohydrates produce glucose, which is used to provide energy. Glucose is stored in the body in fat cells that travel via the bloodstream. People gain weight when there is more fat stored than being used as energy.

Glucose is formed through the consumption of sugar and starch. Namely carbohydrates. The sugars may be in the form of natural sugars from fruit or milk, or they may be formed from processed sugar. Starches like pasta, rice or starchy vegetables like potatoes and corn, form glucose as well. The body breaks down the sugars from these foods into glucose. Glucose and insulin combined to help to carry glucose into the bloodstream so the body can use glucose as energy. The glucose that is not used is stored in the liver and muscles.

In order for the body to supply ketones for use as fuel, the body must use up all the reserves of glucose. In order to do this, there must be a condition of the body of starvation low carbohydrates, passing, or strenuous exercise. A very low carb diet, the production of ketones what her to feel the body and brain.

Ketones are produced from the liver when there is not enough glucose in the body to provide energy. When insulin levels are low, and there is not enough glucose or sugar in the bloodstream, fat is released from fat cells and travels in the blood to the liver. The liver processes the fat into ketones. Ketones are released into the bloodstream to provide fuel for the body and increase the body's metabolism. Ketones are formed under conditions of starvation, fasting, or a diet low in carbohydrates. As ketones are formed, they use the fatty acids, triglycerides, to produce high levels of energy to the muscles, heart, and brain.

Ketones are naturally produced in the body under normal dieting circumstances. The heart and kidney prefer the energy produced from ketones. This is because ketones utilize slow-release energy that is sustained over a long period of time. Glucose energy, which tends to be quick spurts of energy, is less efficient. When ketones are used to fuel the brain, cognitive function can improve and may have a positive impact on brain issues like Parkinson's and dementia. Studies are being done to determine the effectiveness of ketones and ketosis on improving brain function.

How is Insulin Affected by the Keto Diet?

In order to achieve ketosis, insulin production must be minimized. Insulin inhibits the production of ketones. In a normal body, one that doesn't require the introduction of insulin from outside the body, insulin is released from the pancreas, the response to certain foods being consumed. In order to reduce the need for insulin to be released, the diet must be changed so that there are only a few carbs, as few as possible. At the same time, there should only as much protein in the body as it needs in a daily diet.

When a person consumes carbohydrates, the glucose in the carbohydrates is released into the bloodstream. This causes the blood sugar levels to rise in the pancreas to produce insulin into the bloodstream so that the glucose is able to travel through the body and distribute the energy. Leftover glucose that has not been turned into energy becomes stored in fat cells for another time. The stored fat is available then converted to energy when it is called for. For people with type 1 diabetes, the pancreas doesn't make enough insulin to take care of the glucose and blood sugar levels remain high, presenting a dangerous health situation.

Insulin may also be released from the pancreas if there is excess protein in the blood. For this reason, the keto diet stresses the consumption of moderate amounts of protein, and it is important to eat the right combination of protein. The keto diet allows for the consumption of high fat and low protein to provide the optimal combination to enter ketosis. Protein is important for the development of muscle and tissue. Too much protein produces insulin, which inhibits the production of ketones. It is important to provide your body with the correct amount of protein a low amount of carbohydrates. Reducing the grams of carbohydrates eaten minimizes the need for sudden influxes of insulin into the system. In fact, can be reduced over a sustained time period without long-term adverse effects on the body and its health.

Positive Effects of the Keto Diet

The keto diet may have several positive effects on the body. One of the most prominent positive aspects of the keto diet is the ease of sticking to the diet. Successful weight loss plans must be easy to follow for most people to be successful. A low-carb diet may be easy to follow because the keto diet can greatly reduce appetite. If you don't feel hungry, you're more likely to stay on the diet plan. When a person consumes carbohydrates, there is a burst of energy and a feeling of fullness. Unfortunately, these sensations are short-lived because the glucose used to generate energy burns away quickly. This leads to hunger within a short time span. While on keto, the fats will keep you feeling full for a longer period of time. Additionally, as long as you are snacking on items within the plan, there is a lot of room for high-fat items in the diet.

Another good thing about the keto diet, especially in the beginning, you will lose weight. By staying on the plan and following the tenets, you're likely to lose up to twice as much weight at the beginning of a diet as you will with low-fat, low-calorie diets. This is especially true during the first two or three weeks on the diet as the body sheds excess water.

The keto diet reduces the amount of fat stored in the body. The fat loss is made up of visceral fat. Visceral fat is fat that accumulates in the abdomen and tends to attach itself to organs. The keto diet may reduce the fat, which is known to be the most harmful and may reduce the risk of heart disease and type 2 diabetes. These issues are often seen in people who are obese or simply overweight. The visceral fat loss reduces the fat in the most harmful areas of the body and improves overall health in many individuals.

Finally, diets focusing on low carbohydrate consumption will almost always reduce blood sugar levels and improve blood pressure. Carbohydrates increase blood sugar levels. In response to the high blood sugar levels, insulin is produced to regulate blood sugar levels into a normal range. By minimizing the carbohydrates introduced into the bloodstream, your body is not exposed to the spikes of sugar in the bloodstream and effectively reduces the amount of insulin needed to combat the sugar spikes. This will also be instrumental in avoiding the energy lows that are experienced when the carbohydrate energy is burned off. Blood pressure may be positively affected by the keto diet as well. It is important to consume fats that are high in good cholesterol as opposed to bad cholesterol. Good cholesterol is usually present in fats found in plant products like avocados. It has also been found that reducing the consumption of carbohydrates also raises the amount of good cholesterol, HDL, and lowers the amount of bad cholesterol, LDL, in your body.

Negative Effects of Keto

Along with the dramatic change in diet, there may be some negative experiences on the ketogenic diet. One of the more common issues is keto flu. This is a general feeling of fatigue that may accompany entering ketosis. This feeling of tiredness may be accompanied by nausea and upset stomach. It is a common reaction to the body as it adapts to reduced carbohydrates and the switch to getting energy from ketones instead of glucose.

Besides the keto flu, there may also be keto diarrhea. This is likely caused by the gallbladder producing more bile to deal with increased fat consumption. Until the body adjusts to the increased amounts of fat and enters ketosis, diarrhea may be a side effect. Diarrhea may also result from a reduction in the amount of fiber ingested because of a decrease in carbohydrate consumption. The fiber from carbs must be replaced with fiber from low-carb vegetables. This will help mitigate issues with diarrhea resulting from the lack of carbohydrates and, therefore fiber in the diet.

One way to reduce gastrointestinal issues associated with the keto diet is to make sure you drink plenty of water. It is important to stay hydrated and flush out your system. Drinking lots of water helps to remove toxins from the body before they have time to linger in organs and tissues.

The keto diet will precipitate weight loss. Unfortunately, this weight loss may include the reduction of muscle mass as well as fat. This is not ideal, especially for women over 50 in whom muscle mass begins to atrophy naturally. Additionally, reduced muscle mass may change your metabolism because you burn more calories with muscle than fat. This loss of muscle is more likely to happen if you are consuming more fat than protein. The type of fat consumed will be important to retain muscle mass as you lose weight. This will be addressed in a later section of this book.

Keto Mistakes

The most common mistakes revolve around food choices. It is important to maintain correct ratios of fats to proteins. The diet program is subject to fail, and poor health may result in failing to maintain the proper amount of fat. The ketogenic diet is based on using fat to burn as fuel in the body. As a result, the body needs fat to burn. Of course, these need to be good fats that promote increases in HDL cholesterol. This will provide good fuel for the body.

It is important to eat the right fats. Margarine, vegetable oil, canola oil, trans fats, and other light non-viscous plant oils and unhealthy fats should be eliminated from the diet. The fat consumed should be high quality like butter from grass-fed animals, olive oil, monounsaturated oils such as from avocados and coconuts. These are oils and fats are the best options for food and keto. The quality of the fat is important so that it is easily processed and converted to fuel.

Be sure to drink adequate amounts of water when you're on the keto diet. Water will help prevent some of the adverse side effects of the keto diet. It can help with constipation and also help dilute ketones, and acids subject accumulate in the bloodstream. Water is an instrumental factor in avoiding additional weight gain from retention and bloating. You will feel better drinking plenty of water.

Failing to drink adequate amounts of water is a common and unhealthy mistake made by ketogenic dieters. Especially at the beginning of the diet, urination will be frequent. The water needs to be replaced, and you may need to replace electrolytes as well. Make sure to feed your body appropriate nutrients.

When you embark on the keto diet, you may find that you eliminate many processed foods from your diet. These foods use salt as a preservative. Because of this, you will need to replace the salt in your system that you will lose as you drink more water and urinate more frequently. This will help you avoid keto flu or reduce the symptoms of the keto flu.

One of the main mistakes people make on the keto diet is eating too many calories. There is a myth that you can eat whatever you like on the keto diet as long as it is low or no carb and/or high in fat. General life principles are still in effect. If you consume more calories than you burn, you'll gain weight. It is important to maintain vigilance in the number of calories consumed and be sure to eat quality foods containing whole grains and fiber. Though there is room in the diet for keto-friendly snacks, try to avoid processed snacks, which may have more carbohydrates than expected. It is important to review all processed food labels to know the nutritional value of the food you consume.

Chapter 2: Keto for Women Over 50

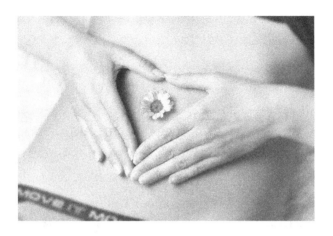

Because of the changes occurring in the bodies of women over 50, it is imperative to look at how the needs of these women are different than younger women and men. During menopause, hormones shift in women, and these changes make it necessary to make some adjustments to their lifestyle in general, and diet in particular.

General Nutritional Needs for Women Over 50

As a woman enters her fifties, it becomes necessary to make modifications to the diet to be healthy. This is because of changes in hormones and metabolism. There is a decrease in muscle mass. To offset this change, there is a need to increase the amount of protein in the diet. At the same time, bone density decreases, making it necessary to increase the amount of vitamin D and calcium consumed in order to maintain adequate bone density as the body ages. All this, combined with a reduction in the number of calories needed to fuel the body, makes it necessary to modify diet as a woman enters postmenopausal years. These natural changes to the body make changes to the diet necessary as a woman ages.

Also, as women age, their ability to discern thirstiness may diminish. Water consumption is still an important factor in the health of a woman. Because it is harder to determine thirst as you surpass your 50th year, it is essential that you consume 8 to 9 8 oz glasses of water each day. Drink more in the winter in hot weather and when exercising. While you are drinking more water, it may serve to curb your appetite. This is good because you will need to lower your caloric intake from what you may be accustomed to. this happens when you are finding new aches and pains and slowing down your exercise regime. Exercise may be less intense as you make modifications to coincide with your age and decreases in mobility. This is because you are not as flexible and may be experiencing inflammation in your joints. While these are all relatively normal signs of aging, the decrease in physical activity may cause additional problems in the form of weight gain.

This may be a good time to eliminate processed foods and sugar from your diet. Dietary fiber is the key to avoiding constipation. Studies show that women over 50 may be up to seven times more likely to suffer from constipation than men of a similar age. Failure to consume enough dietary fiber can result in small, hard stool. It is beneficial to consume dietary fiber, which is found in whole grains, and food is made from whole grains, as well as fruits and vegetables. The foods move through intestines easily and make solid stool that moves through the intestines quickly and efficiently. The dietary fiber in these foods may help in lowering bad cholesterol (LDL) levels in adults. This may have a positive effect on heart health as well. Since estrogen levels in women are also decreasing, the female body begins to lose the positive effect estrogen has on the heart and blood vessels. This is another impact of menopause. Consuming adequate amounts of dietary fiber may help to improve heart health.

Gentler Approach to Keto for Women Over 50

Women over 50 may want to modify their keto approach by increasing the daily carbohydrates to 100 to 150 g each day. They may also want to increase the protein from 25% to 30% of the diet. The remaining amount of food will be fat. The increased carbohydrates provide less distress to hormones and metabolism and put less stress on the body while adjusting to a diet low in carbohydrates. The increase in protein is to offset the body's tendency to lose muscle mass as women age. Additionally, the carbs will provide energy to exercise. The metabolism of women typically slow as women age. The increase in carbs and protein may allow women over 50 to forgo the sluggish feelings and allow enough energy to exercise while on the diet. This will improve overall health.

Carbohydrates in your diet should come from whole grains or high-quality carbs like pumpkins, carrots, spaghetti squash, and small quantities of butternut squash. Foods that grow below the ground have higher carbohydrate content. If you feel like you need to sneak them into your diet, it should be small amounts per serving. They add variety and flavor to your diet, but they must be used in moderation. Even with a few extra carbs in your diet, you should be able to enter ketosis. The same is true for protein. The body may not enter ketosis as quickly, but the effects of the changes will not be as jarring to your body and the internal system of operation.

The keto diet stresses the importance of high fiber low carb food. Be sure to include leafy greens and healthy oils in the diet. The leafy greens will help avoid gastrointestinal issues during keto. They contain the fiber lost with the reduction of carbohydrates. Many vegetables contain carbohydrates, so be aware of the amount you are eating and stay within your macros. Some of the vegetables have fiber and no carbohydrates, but others, like cauliflower and jicama, have carbs. You must remember to count them in your daily totals. Green leafy vegetables have protein that must be added as well. Overall, it is best to get your fiber from vegetables to keep you energized and lessen the effects of keto flu and keto diarrhea, as well as constipation.

Tracking and Macros

Macronutrients are found in every food. They are the nutrients that fuel the body. Carbohydrates, proteins, and fats are included in the calories consumed and should be tracked while on the keto diet. The information needed is on the nutritional value label found on foods. Accurately measure individual portions to be sure to have accurate nutritional information. These nutrients being tracked are typically called "macros" which is a shortened version of the word macronutrient. This book specifies the macros that you need to know for a ketogenic diet plan. By making adjustments to the SKD and HPKD, a gentler keto plan may be created in order to fit the needs of women over 50.

First, we will look at the carbohydrates. You will be counting net carbs. Grams of net carbs are determined by subtracting the grams of dietary fiber and the grams of sugar alcohols from the grams of total carbohydrates. Dietary fiber does not release insulin into the body. The same is true of sugar alcohols. As a result, you will be able to eat more nutritionally dense foods and may satisfy your food cravings and hunger.

Next, we will look at fats. You will be eating 60 to 75% of your food as fat. This allows for a wide variety of foods, like bacon and pork rinds, to be included in your diet. Avocado, nuts, and other foods will be included in your diet as well. Because you will be eating food that is not processed, it will be important to eat healthy fats including oil derived from natural food sources like avocado oil and coconut oil. High-quality butter and ghee will also be good sources of fat.

When we start to consider proteins, proteins do not need to be lean meats. In fact, the proteins included in keto should not be lean but should be high in fat so that you consume appropriate amounts of fat. The keto diet is only effective when there is a high amount of fat consumed.

Now, let's start calculating the macros. In order to calculate the grams of net carbohydrates to include in your daily diet, it is important to determine your body weight and then your percentage of body fat. To do this, weigh yourself. After determining your weight, divide your body weight by your height in inches and square height in inches squared. Multiply that by 703 and you will have your BMI, or body mass index.

Lbs/height in inches, squared, times 703=BMI. So, in actuality, if you are a 5-foot 6-inch woman weighing 200 lb that's, $200/66^2$ x 703=32.28. The BMI is 32.28.

Then calculate your body fat percentage. (1.2 x BMI) + (.23 * age) - 5.4 equals body fat percentage. When we plug in the BMI from our female example,

(1.2 * 32.28) + (.23*55) - 5.4 =45.98

So, the body fat percentage is 45.98%. Now that you have your body fat percentage take your body fat percentage and multiply it by your body weight. 45.98% x 200 lb. That equals 91.96 lbs of body fat. Subtract the body fat from your weight and you have your LBM (Lean Body Mass). So, 200 - 91.96 equals 108.04. The LBM is 108.04.

Now, it's time to determine the number of macronutrients to eat each day.
We can start with the calculation for protein. There are .8 grams per pound of lean body mass. In our example, .8* 108.04 equals 84 grams. This is equal to 346 calories because there are 4 calories in each gram of protein. In our example, 20% of the calories the daily calories will be from protein. Therefore, 346 calories/.20 equals 1730 calories per day.

The total calories are 1730 calories per day.

To determine the number of carbohydrates, let's look at the number of carbohydrates in a gentler keto. 10% of the daily calories will come from carbs. 10% of 1730 calories is 173 calories. If you divide 173 calories by 4 (there are 4 calories in each carbohydrate), you will have 43.25g of carbohydrates as your daily allowance.

The remaining calories for each day will be fat calories:

     346 Calories, Protein
  86.50g   20%

                       +173 Calories, Carbohydrate
    43.25g   10%
                    519 Calories   of Protein and Carbs
                   -1730 (Total Daily Calories)
                   1211 Calories, Fat
    134.56g   70%

There are 9 calories in each fat gram. 1,211 calories/9 calories = 134.56g of fat for each day, or 70% of your daily calorie intake.

These macros will change as your BMI and LBM change. Make sure you adjust your macros every four or five weeks while you're losing weight so that your macros are accurate. You will want to record what you are eating and review your success in weight loss. This will allow you to track how your body is reacting to food combinations. Each body is different, and it is important to see how you feel when you are eating different foods and combinations of foods as your approach ketosis. Be sure you're eating whole grains and getting fiber through leafy green vegetables. You will also want to be very familiar with nutrition labels to be sure you're not consuming hidden carbohydrates without realizing you are doing so.

Fasting Over 50

Intermittent fasting (IF) is sometimes used to lose weight in combination with a keto diet. It has been an effective way to lose weight for some women. After menopause, some women may gain weight for seemingly no reason. It may be that the general stressors in life cause a new source of weight gain because of cortisol, which may trigger your body to store fat in the abdominal region. Intermittent fasting may be a viable weight loss solution if there is an excess of cortisol being released into your system. The most common forms of IF are 5:2, 12:12, and 16:8.

For the 5:2 fast, one eats normally for 5 days and fasts for 2 days. The two days are not actually a complete fast, but drastically reduced the caloric intake of around 500 calories plus liquids like water and sugar-free drinks. During the 5 days, any foods are allowed to be eaten.

The 12:12 fast is 12 hours of fasting and 12 hours of eating. During the 12 hours of eating, it is important to eat regular meals and snacks. The calorie consumption should be consistent with a normal caloric intake of 2000 recommended calories per day. Make sure the calories are good calories and avoid empty carbohydrates and unhealthy fats.

The same is true for the 16/8 intermediate fast. Fasting lasts for 16 hours. During the 8 hour period, eat at least two meals each day and a snack, maybe two snacks. These meals should be thoughtful meals that do not have excess calories and or carbohydrates.

Fasting, in combination with the keto diet, can promote more rapid weight loss. Fasting may be a way to reach ketosis more quickly. After achieving ketosis, if you've not been intermittently fasting, it may be helpful to introduce fasting to reinitiate weight loss. If you're at a plateau, and you have already been fasting, it may be helpful to begin a different form of fasting. This may trigger new weight loss while in ketosis.

Keto Diet for Longevity

Though there is no absolute proof, recent studies have shown a correlation between the ketogenic diet and a longer, better life. The caveat is, the protein used to replace carbohydrates should be vegetable and plant-based proteins. Additionally, the carbohydrates consumed should be complex. Natural foods are encouraged, and processed carbohydrates, like white bread, sugary carbohydrates and drinks should be avoided. Unhealthy fats should be avoided as well. The fats consumed should be derived from plants to be healthier. This includes avocado oil, olive oil, and coconut oil. The fiber found in bread and other grains eliminated in a keto diet must be replaced with vegetable fiber so that your body continues to be nourished in an appropriate manner. By continuing to eat an appropriate amount of fiber and nutrients, the keto diet can be a healthy and effective weight loss plan.

Some studies are reporting that low-carb diets, including ketogenic diets, are reducing lifespans. The problem with many of these studies is that they are uncontrolled and rely on subjects who report their actions after a period of time has passed. The periods of contact may extend beyond a year or more. To this date, the scientific study of low carbohydrate and ketogenic diets is limited to the study of mice who have been introduced to the ketogenic lifestyle. The mice in the study became less agitated, move about easier, and seem to have better mobility. The lifespan of these mice has also increased.

Overall, it is believed that the improvements in health and evidence of increased longevity through the ketogenic diet are the result of proper study and may be factually true. The reduction of insulin spikes and general weight loss have positive effects on heart health and improve cardiovascular function, especially for people losing weight during and after middle age. With a reduction in inflammation of the body and joints, decreased pain, and increased mobility, people feel better while on the keto diet. Many dieters are able to exercise more as well and are able to exercise on a regular basis. They are able to do all the things people are told will increase their health and lifespan. Health is improved in a way that does go a long way in improving the quality, as well as the longevity of life.

Exercise for Women Over 50 in Support of Keto

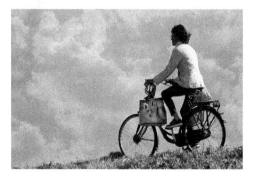

While you are on the keto diet, if your goal is to lose weight, you will be thinking of exercising to assist your body in shedding excess pounds. The problem will be that you may not feel like exercising, especially at the beginning. As your body transitions to ketosis, keto flu may cause feelings of lethargy. When taking all this into account, there are still good reasons for women over the age of 50 to exercise while on the keto diet.

One of the primary reasons exercise is important is the loss of muscle mass women experience as they grow older. In order to combat this loss, exercise is an ideal way to strengthen your body and retain muscle. When we look at what exercises to do, they should be limited, at the beginning of the keto diet, to strengthening and endurance exercises. Even if you are used to strenuous exercise, it is better, until your body adapts to ketosis, to pare down your workouts to a level that does not tire quickly. Your endurance will probably be affected by the switch from using carbs as energy to using fat as energy. It is important not to deplete your energy stores so that your body starts to glean energy from muscles.

As your body enters ketosis, you may find that you feel better, your joints are not as achy, and you're ready to exercise more. Your body is likely to be in better shape than it was, and you will want to capitalize on your new healthy state. This will give you the opportunity to increase your exercises as you enjoy the benefits of the keto diet and ketosis. One should always start out slowly and increase exertion over time so that your muscles are not exhausted and you feel good even while working out. Be sure to drink lots of water during workouts and you may need to replenish nutrients after working out to replace those lost due to sweat and muscle fatigue.

For women over 50, it may be a good idea to limit your exercises to those that do not add a lot of stress to the body. The ability to move around better is often a positive side effect of the keto diet. This will allow you to strengthen and tone your muscles. Start off slowly and add to your exercises as your body recovers and adapts to the keto diet. Be sure to listen to your body as you worked out, and if you feel tired or your muscles feel strained, stop working out for that time period. Your body will tell you how much it can endure. Switching to a keto diet will cause some strain on your body, to begin with, so take time to build up to a good workout while you are on the diet.

While you're on the keto diet, it will be important to do strength-building exercises and low-intensity workouts in order to continue to burn fat while you're exercising. When you switch over to a high-intensity workout, you will be burning carbohydrates. Because there are only a few carbohydrates in your system, it is difficult to sustain a workout high-intensity level. So, assuming that you are an average person is on the keto diet for weight loss purposes, it will be best to maintain low-intensity workouts. The best are cardio workouts like walking and jogging, as well as strength workouts such as yoga. Yoga is always a good source of exercise as we age. It is a way to strengthen the core and improve balance and muscle tone. If you are using weights in your workout, you should use lighter weights, lighter than you are used to. Increase the repetition so that it is a low-intensity workout. Again, low-intensity workouts burn fat. If weight loss is the goal, you want to lose fat. So, low-intensity exercise should be your goal.

Tips and Tricks for Ketogenic Weight Loss

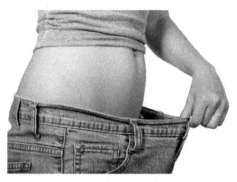

Now that we've gone over the ketogenic diet and all the things involved with being on the ketogenic diet, it is a good time to look at some tips and tips and tricks to being successful on the keto diet.

1. **Limit your carbohydrate intake.** The whole point of the ketogenic diet is to substantially reduce your consumption of carbohydrates. Even if practicing a gentler keto, as recommended for women over 50, you still need to be mindful of the carbs you are consuming. Be sure not to eat hidden carbohydrates that are often found in processed foods. Be wary of "lite" and "low fat" foods. They often get their flavor from sugar. Sugar is, of course, low in fat. On the contrary, sugar is high in carbohydrates. It is a good idea to eliminate almost all forms of sugar on the ketogenic diet. Don't let your carb intake exceed 10%.
2. **Introduce coconut oil into your diet.** Coconut oil is full of nutrients that metabolize quickly in your

liver and is converted to energy right away. Consuming coconut oil may help you reach ketosis faster. It's a really easy way to motivate your body to be in ketosis.

3. **Exercise.** It is important to maintain your muscle mass, perhaps increase your muscle mass. Make sure that you're doing exercises involving strength and endurance. Keep the exercises a low-intensity level so that you're burning fat, and not using carbohydrates.

4. **Eat enough fat.** You have to be sure, while you are on the ketogenic diet, that you are eating enough fat. The fat you eat is going to be converted into energy. You need to have enough fat in your body to supply energy to your brain, organs, and muscles to sustain yourself and your activities. Additionally, make sure that you are using your macros to decide what to eat, and that you recalculate your macros from time to time. Be sure you know what you're eating and that you're meeting your nutrient needs, including fat, for each day.

5. **Track your food.** Keep a record of your food consumption. Be sure to add in all the "bits and bites" that pass your lips. You know, the food that you test while cooking? That corner of a cookie you broke off as a little nibble? Record everything you eat so that you know you're meeting your macros. Read labels to make sure you know what you're eating. This book will include a guide on raw foods and meats so that you can calculate how many nutrients are in the foods

that you are eating after you have eliminated processed foods from your diet.
6. **Intermittent fasting.** As previously reviewed in this book, intermittent fasting can be a good way to get into ketosis more quickly. The body will adjust to getting energy from fat molecules in your body, and you may enter ketosis more quickly. You may also use intermittent fasting while you're in ketosis to lose more weight.
7. **Control your protein intake.** If you have been on previous weight loss plans, you are probably adhering to low-fat, high protein diets. Because we are following macros, it is important to eat the correct amount of protein. Do not eat too much protein, because you will throw off your fat or carbohydrates. Eating too little protein will cause your body to lose muscle mass. On the ketogenic diet, we will we want to adhere to the correct ratios of proteins, fats, and carbohydrates in order to optimize weight loss and fat loss in the body.
8. **Drink lots of water.** Water is essential to the body, and you will lose a lot of water on the ketogenic diet. The water must be replaced, especially after exercise. You may also want to take a mineral supplement or drink water with electrolytes so that your chemical balance is maintained after working out. Replacing the water lost through sweat and urination will keep your body working properly. You will feel better if you stay hydrated throughout your ketogenic diet.

9. **Reduce your stress.** Try to remain stress-free during your ketogenic diet. As discussed, cortisol levels in your body will cause your body to retain fat, especially in the abdominal region. You want to be sure that your body is not working at cross purposes. Stress may trigger your body to store fat in reaction to stress while you are trying to lose fat on your ketogenic diet. Make sure you incorporate activities in your day to reduce your stress level. Some people find yoga is a good way to relax. Others use hobbies as a way to relieve tension and reduce stress.
10. **Get lots of sleep.** Make sure you get enough sleep. Each night your body needs 7 to 9 hours of sleep. Sleep allows us time to rejuvenate our bodies and store up energy. Be sure to do things that promote a sleep-inducing atmosphere. Turn off the lights, limit the use of electronics and like computers and smartphones within 30 minutes of sleeping and refrain from using them in bed. Turn off the television and prepare your room and your body for sleep. Try to maintain a consistent schedule of sleep. These things may make it easier to get to sleep. People on the keto diet have reported better sleep, reduced snoring, and waking up refreshed. Set the scene so that you will be able to benefit from better sleep on the diet.
11. **Know your goals.** Before you start the ketogenic diet, determine your goals, and write down the reasons why you're on the ketogenic diet. If you want to lose weight, also note why you want to lose weight.

This is important, so you can always refer back to the reasons you began the diet. It is sometimes helpful to remember what your goals are and why you want to meet those goals. This will be a good touchstone when you want to reach for a cookie or a sugary drink. Make sure you have that goal handy so that when you're feeling weak, you can remind yourself of your goals are and be determined to stick to them.

Chapter 3: Keto Food and Ketosis

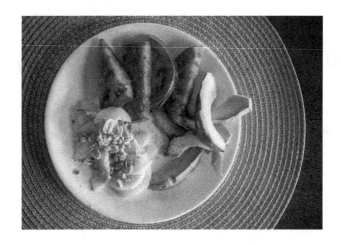

After determining what the macros look like and how many calories you should be consuming each day, you will need to decide what to eat. There are many options that are keto-friendly, so finding something to eat will probably not be a problem. There will have to be decisions made regarding food quality and food quantity.

Food Quality

It is better to eat foods that are of high quality on the keto diet. The right chemical makeup of your food assists in a successful journey to ketosis. Because you will be using food to fuel your body, it is important to eat the best quality food available to get the key nutrients you will need to sustain your brain and body health.

Grass-fed meat from grazing animals is suggested because it tends to be higher in omega-3 fatty acids. Cage-free poultry and eggs are also preferred on keto. Butter should be of high quality with high-fat content. Grass-fed meats clan to have fewer calories than grain-fed needs. Additionally, the grain-fed to conventionally bred animals often contains growth hormone which will be passed to you when you eat it. The grass-fed meat products are healthier and lower in calories. There can be up to five times more omega-3 fatty acids in grass-fed beef than grain-fed. Grass-fed beef also contains electrolytes. Electrolytes control nerve pulses and muscle contractions. They leave your body through urination, which will be more frequent while on the keto diet. Electrolytes need to be replaced to keep your body in balance. Grass-fed beef will help to restore magnesium, potassium, and sodium and assist in minimizing the effects of the keto flu.

Eating organic vegetables and fruit, though not required, may be considered optimal when you are making an effort to eat the cleanest and healthiest food. Whether an item is organic or conventional, the keto effects are the same. The benefit of eating organic food is a reduction in the amount of chemicals and pesticide residue. The nutritional characteristics are the same and hold true whether the produce is fresh or frozen. No matter what, be sure to cleanse your produce and your preparation area regularly. Inspect the produce for pests and debris to be sure the washing and soaking have done a good job, especially when you are eating raw fruits and vegetables. Remember to concentrate on dark green vegetables and try to get the freshest possible. Good quality produce will provide good nutrients to fuel your body.

Foods to Eat

The variety of foods you can eat on the keto diet is vast. After determining the macros to follow, you can find foods that fit into the macros for your daily food. It will be important to have enough nutrients to sustain yourself while on the diet and to be able to safely stay on the keto diet.

Fats

Your daily consumption of fats will be around 70% of your food intake. This needs to be high-quality fat that stays in your system to be used as energy. These are typically found in fats that are the result of raw foods and animals.

Some of the best fats for keto are:

Hard Cheeses
Nuts like almonds, walnuts, pecans, and macadamia
Seeds from sunflowers, pumpkins, chia, flaxseed and hemp hearts
Natural oils like olive oil and coconut oil
Cacao of at least 85% cacao. This must be unsweetened and unprocessed chocolate
Poultry, especially dark meat
Fatty fish
Whole eggs, especially the yolks

Whole milk produces like whole milk mozzarella and ricotta

Cheese

When we look at high-fat foods, cheese tops the list. It is high in fat and has no carbohydrates. Unfortunately, cheese contains a lot of calories, along with unhealthy saturated fats. When you are consuming cheese, be mindful of the amount you eat. Some cheese is a healthy snack and a good alternative to chips and sugary snack items. Small amounts of cheese in your diet, a few ounces daily, will help you control your hunger because it is filling. It has also been found that calcium in cheese may have a positive effect on blood pressure and cholesterol. Consumption of cheese has also been found to increase muscle mass.

Nuts

As you choose which nuts you're going to eat on keto, be sure to take note of the net carbs. Some nuts have more fat than others, and some have more calories and carbohydrates than others. Choose nuts that will fit well in your macros. Because of the high calories and carbs eat nuts in moderation. They may also have a significant amount of protein when eating a large quantity. Be sure you are adhering to your protein macros as well as your carbohydrate macros.

Seeds

The good thing about seeds in relation to keto is that the carbohydrates are mostly offset by fiber. That makes the net carbohydrates friendly for keto. Seeds tend to be high in fat and contain some protein. They often contain harmful omega-6 fatty acids, though. You can benefit from the healthy concentration of nutrients in seeds, but eating them sprouted. In order to sprout seeds, simply germinate the seeds between two wet paper towels and leave them to sit for 2 to 8 days. Make sure your paper towel remains moist. Eventually, the stem will sprout from the seed. It's still high in nutrients but easier to digest.

Oils

Oils can be your best cooking aid in the keto diet. They must be able to burn at high temperatures to be most effective for cooking. It is important to use unsaturated fats to provide the most heart-healthy oils. The polyunsaturated oils will be a good addition to the fats consumed on a keto like nut oils and avocado oils. These will assist you in achieving a healthy, effective keto diet. Avocado oil, sesame oil, coconut oil, and olive oil have essential qualities to aid in digestion and nutrient absorption. Also, coconut oil speeds up metabolism.

Meat/Fish/Eggs/Dairy

Unprocessed meats do not contain carbohydrates, and many are high in fat. Grass-fed meats are better than grain-fed but watch the portion size. Be careful not to exceed the protein requirements in your daily macros. Fish is good, especially fish high in fat like salmon. Avoid the breading, which has carbohydrates. Again, wild-caught fish is better. It is fed naturally off of foods fish are accustomed to eating. This is Lloyd's the chance that growth hormones and antibiotics may be included in the feed from farm fat raised fish. Along the same lines, try to stick to cage-free pasture-raised eggs in the hopes of avoiding chemical additives that might reduce the quality of the food you are consuming. The same is true for milk. Milk and dairy products should be organic to avoid growth hormones and antibiotics that may be found in conventional Foods today. Meat fish eggs and dairy are high in fat; I can be a good source of the fat you need to consume on the keto diet.

Proteins

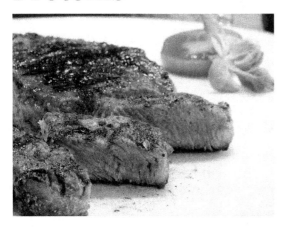

Protein will make up 20% of your daily food intake. It is important not to exceed your protein macros. Be sure you're making good decisions regarding your protein if a person that you are including your diet. It will be consuming a lot of fat, which may contain a lot of protein. So you have to be sure to combine your fat macros with your protein macros when you're setting up your meal plan for the day.

Some of the proteins that you will be eating that are most efficient are:

Salmon
Mackerel
Tuna
Sardines
Eggs
Greek yogurt
Shrimp
Chicken thighs
Peanuts
Pistachios
Almonds
Soybeans (edamame)
Nut butters

The goal of the keto diet is not to eat low-fat proteins. Luckily, there are many high-fat proteins available for consumption. Many times, you will be able to satisfy your fat macros and protein macros with the same food items. Watch your calories, and be sure to incorporate your snack foods into your protein count. Be mindful that green leafy vegetables also contain protein.

It is important to consume enough protein so that carbohydrates in your body do not use muscle to convert to energy. Conversely, too much protein can cause muscle tissue to break down and turn into sugar because of the lack of carbohydrates available on a low-carb diet. Eat the right amount of protein, and don't forget about adding in the protein found snacks and vegetables, especially cream leafy ones when considering your protein macros.

Fish

Some of the best foods for protein on keto are fatty proteins found in salmon, mackerel, and sardines. These proteins are high in fat and omega-3 fatty acids. Fresh fish is higher in omega-3 fatty acid than canned fish, but if you are going to eat fish protein, make sure it is high in fat. This is an efficient way to consume protein and fat that will be converted to energy.

Eggs

Some studies indicate that people who include dairy in their diet have less hunger, and the consumption of dairy may inhibit the production of cortisol, and therefore, the resulting abdominal fat. Full-fat dairy is high in calories, so be sure not to over-consume. It is common for conventional milk and dairy products to contain growth hormones. Dairy from grass-fed animals and organic dairy products are recommended. Aside from the hormones, conventional dairy products do not have as high levels of omega-3 fatty acids, which have anti-inflammatory qualities and promote joint health. Dairy contains a lot of protein. If you're eating meat protein, you should be especially cognizant of the amount of dairy that you're eating so you do not exceed your protein macros. Egg whites are lower in calories and contain the protein of the egg. The egg yolks contain the fat of eggs. If you're going to eat meat and eggs and you have consumed enough fat for the daily macro, you may be able to eat the white instead of the yolks without adding additional fat. The yolk also carries the bulk of calories from eggs and egg whites have very few calories.

Nuts/Nut Butters/Soybeans

Nuts and soybeans (edamame) make excellent snack foods on keto. Eating good quality protein and protein-filled snacks, especially after exercising, may assist your body in building muscle. Snacks should be kept small. They should simply be a means to curb your hunger pains. That is why a quick snack of nuts is ideal. They contain some proteins, some fats, and some carbohydrates. Count the nuts you select to be sure you don't eat too many carbs. Carefully measure the serving size of your snack. Since nuts are small, it is easy to think that eating a few extra nuts here and there won't matter. Whether this is true depends on the nut. That's a good way to add moderate levels of protein to your diet and to adjust your protein macros for the day.

Carbohydrates

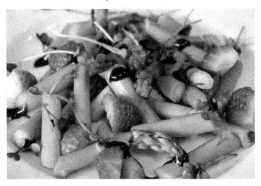

So far, it has been stressed to eat more fat, the correct amount of protein, and now, it is time for carbohydrates. Eat fewer carbohydrates. Consume 10% of your daily food in the form of carbohydrates. This is the crux of the ketogenic diet. Normally, carbohydrates are limited to 5% of the daily calories eaten. In doing the gentle keto, the carbohydrates are increased to 10%. Whether 5% or 10%, be sure to minimize the number of carbohydrates in your diet. Also, try to make the carbohydrates of good quality that will burn off quickly so that your body moves quickly to burning fat.

There are many no-carb options available when eating fats and protein. What is needed to add to your diet are vegetables. Produce has nutrients and vitamins that your body needs, so they should be included in your diet. Be sure to incorporate foods that have valuable nutrients such as vegetables and berries into your diet. These are low in carbohydrates. Some of the vegetables and fruits should be used more sparingly than others. Look at green leafy vegetables and vegetables that grow above the ground as low carbohydrate options to provide healthy options that will not add fat. Vegetables that grow underground like carrots and potatoes tend to have more sugar content and are higher in carbohydrates. Here is a list of fruits and vegetables that are good to eat on keto (Yes), should be excluded from your keto diet (No), and fruits and vegetables that may be eaten occasionally (Maybe):

Yes	No	Maybe
Asparagus	Apples	Artichokes
Avocado	Apricots	Blackberries
Bell peppers	Bananas	Blueberries
Bok choy	Beets	Broccoli
Broccoli rabe	Cantaloupe	Brussels sprouts

Cauliflower	Cherries	Carrots
Celery	Corn	Coconut meat
Cucumbers	Cranberries	Eggplant
Greens	Dried fruit	Fennel
Mushrooms	Grapes	Ginger
Radishes	Leek	Honeydew
Sprouts (alfalfa, bean)	Mango	Jicama
Summer squash (zucchini, yellow)	Oranges	Kiwi
	Papaya	Lemon juice
	Peaches	Lime juice

YES	NO	Maybe
	Pears	Olives (black, green)
	Pineapple	Onions
	Plums	Raspberries
	Potatoes	Rhubarb
	Sweet potatoes	Spaghetti Squash
	Watermelon	Strawberries
	Winter Squash	Tomatoes

Green leafy vegetables like kale, spinach, collard greens, mustard greens, romaine lettuce, and arugula are low in net carbohydrates and high in vitamins and nutrients. These items should be integrated into your keto diet so that you are sure to be receiving enough nutrients for a healthy diet. Though not "free" foods, because they have carbohydrates of varying amounts, they are items that you can eat easily and are necessary for soluble fibers. Eating your vegetables may help to stave off constipation. Leafy greens and other vegetables where you eat the parts of the plant exposed to pesticides are better if purchased organic. If you do not purchase organically-grown products, be sure to clean your leafy greens, even if it is packaged and says it is pre-washed.

The items in the "NO" column are very high in sugar and carbohydrates. Eating them will easily knock you out of ketosis. Even though some of the items are vegetables, root vegetables have a lot of sugar. Also, most fruits are not allowed on keto.

Avocados are also in the carbohydrate section of foods. Basically, avocados are the keto superfood. They are high in fat and protein, low in carbohydrates. They have good nutritional value.

The only fruits that are really allowed on the keto diet are berries. Because you eat the seed, they are higher in fiber. They tend to be the lowest carbohydrates in the fruit families. Avocados are a nice addition because they are high in fat and high in fiber, as well as low in carbohydrates. Other fruits are very high in sugar. In fact, two apples can be your entire carbohydrate macro for a day.

If you feel you need to eat starchy, Foods replace those foods with cauliflower. Cauliflower has two grams of net carbs per cup. Potatoes have 26 grams per cup and rice has 45 grams per cup. These carb counts have been a reason for the increasing popularity of riced cauliflower. Luckily, it is available frozen and packaged in the fresh produce section of most grocery stores, so its not necessary to waste time operating your food processor.

Some other vegetables that you may eat on your keto diet are asparagus, green beans, mushrooms, tomatoes, eggplant, cucumber, bell pepper, celery, and cabbage. Onions are also included on the keto diet mainly because they are eaten sparingly, and the amount of onions in a recipe is spread out among many servings in a dish.

Adding a variety of vegetables into your keto diet may help you to feel better and also help you avoid some of the negative effects of the keto diet like constipation and possibly the keto flu. It is important to maintain adequate vitamins and nutrients in your diet, and vegetables and berries fit the bill. Vegetables such as spinach, kale, collard greens, turnip greens, romaine lettuce, and certain cabbages are foods that you can eat without affecting ketosis. They are high in nutrients and low in net carbs.

Below is a generalized list of foods and their nutritional content. Check the entire nutritional content of foods and maintain the correct serving sizes, so you do not exceed the calories allowed with your keto macros.

Nutritional Food List

Food	Serving Size	Net Carb	Protein	Fat	Calories
Alfalfa sprouts	1/2 cup	1g	1.5g	0g	15
Almond butter (w/o salt)	1 Tbls	1.5g	3.5g	9g	98
Almond meal/flour	1/4 cup	3g	6g	11g	150
Almonds	23 nuts	2.5g	6g	14g	164
Artichoke	1/2 medium	3.5g	1.7g	0g	32
Artichoke hearts, canned	1 heart	0.5g	0g	1.5g	15
Food	**Serving Size**	**Net Carb**	**Protein**	**Fat**	**Calories**

Artichoke hearts, marinated	4 pieces	2g	0g	6g	60
Arugula	1 cup	0.5g	0.5g	0g	5
Asparagus	6 spears	2g	2g	0g	20
Avocado	1/2 fruit	3.5g	3.5g	15g	182
Bamboo shoots	1/2 cup	1g	1g	0g	12
Beans, green	1/2 cup	2g	1g	0g	16
Beet greens	1/2 cup	2g	2g	0g	19
Blackberries, fresh	1/4 cup	4g	0.5g	0.2g	15
Blackberries, frozen	1/4 cup	4g	0.5g	0.2g	24
Blue cheese	1 oz.	0.7g	6g	8g	100

Food	Serving Size	Net Carb	Protein	Fat	Calories
Bok choy	1/2 cup	0.5g	1.3g	0g	10
Boston/bibb lettuce	1 cup	0g	1g	0g	7
Brazil nuts	5 nuts	1g	3.5g	17g	165
Brie	1 oz.	0.1g	6g	8g	95
Broccoflower	1/2 cup	1g	1g	0g	10
Broccoli	1/2 cup	3g	2g	0g	27
Broccoli florets	1/2 cup	1g	1g	0g	10
Broccoli rabe	1/2 cup	0.3g	3.3g	0.5g	28
Brussels sprouts	1/4	2g	1g	0g	14

	cup				
Butter or ghee	1 Tbls	0g	0.12g	11.5g	102
Cabbage, green	1/2 cup	2.5g	1g	0g	17
Cabbage, red	1/2 cup	3g	1g	0g	22
Cabbage, savoy	1/2 cup	2g	1.3g	0g	17
Cashew butter (w/o salt)	1 Tbls	4g	3g	8g	94
Cashews	1/4 cup	9g	4g	12g	150
Cauliflower	1/2 cup	1g	1g	0.3g	14
Cauliflower florets	1/2 cup	2g	1g	0g	13
Celery	1 stalk	0.5g	0g	0g	6

Food	Serving Size	Net Carb	Protein	Fat	Calories
Celery	1/2 cup	1.8g	0.5g	0g	14
Chard, swiss	1/2 cup	1.5g	2g	0g	18
Chayote	1/2 cup	2g	0.5g	0.4g	19
Cheddar or colby	1 oz.	1g	6.5g	9.5g	115
Food	**Serving Size**	**Net Carb**	**Protein**	**Fat**	**Calories**
Cherries, fresh, pitted	1/4 cup	5g	0.4g	0.1g	24
Chicory greens	½ cup	0.5g	0g	0g	3
Chinese cabbage	1/2 cup	0.5g	0.5g	0g	5
Chives	1 Tbls	0g	0.1g	0g	1
Coconut, shredded,	1/4 cup	1g	1g	7g	71

unsweetened					
Coconut butter	1 Tbls	1.5g	1g	10.5g	105
Coconut oil	1 Tbls	0g	0g	13.47g	121
Collard greens	1/2 cup	1.5g	2.5g	1g	31
Cottage cheese (2% fat)	1/2 cup	5g	12g	2.5g	92
Cranberries, raw, chopped	1/4 cup	2g	0.1g	0g	13
Cream cheese	2 Tbls	0.6g	2g	10g	100
Cucumber (with peel)	1/2 cup, sliced	1.7g	0.3g	0g	8
Daikon radish	1/2 cup	1g	0.4g	0g	9
Dandelion greens	1/2 cup	2g	1g	0.3g	17

Food	Serving Size	Net Carb	Protein	Fat	Calories
Eggplant	1/2 cup	3g	1g	0g	17
Endive	1/2 cup	0g	0.3g	0g	4
Food	**Serving Size**	**Net Carb**	**Protein**	**Fat**	**Calories**
Escarole	1/2 cup	0.3g	1g	0g	14
Fennel, bulb	1/2 cup	1.5g	0.5g	0g	13
Fennel, bulb	1/2 cup	2g	0.5g	0g	13
Flaxseed oil	1 Tbls	0g	0.01g	13.6g	120
Goat cheese (soft)	1 oz.	0g	5g	6g	75
Gouda	1 oz.	0.6g	7g	8g	100
Greens, mixed	1 cup	0.5g	0.5g	0g	5

Food	Serving Size	Net Carb	Protein	Fat	Calories
Hazelnuts	12 nuts	1.5g	2.5g	10g	106
Hearts of palm	1 heart	0.5g	1g	0.2g	9
Heavy whipping cream	1 Tbls	0.4g	0.4g	5.4g	51
Heavy whipping cream	1/2 cup	1.6g	1.7g	22g	204
Iceberg lettuce	1 cup	1g	0.7g	0g	10
Jicama	1/2 cup	2g	0.5g	0g	23
Kale	1/2 cup	2.5g	1g	0g	18
Kohlrabi	1/4 cup	2.5g	1g	0g	12
Lard/Dripping	1 Tbls	0g	0g	12.8g	115

Leeks	1/2 cup	3.5g	0.5g	0g	16
Loganberries, frozen	1/4 cup	3g	0.6g	0.1g	20
Loose-leaf lettuce	1 cup	2g	0.5g	0g	8
Macadamia butter	1 Tbls	1g	2g	10g	97
Macadamias	6 nuts	0.8g	1g	11g	102
Mayonnaise	1 Tbls	0.08g	0.13g	10.33g	94
Melon, cantaloupe	1/4 cup	3g	0.4g	0.1g	15
Melon, honeydew	1/4 cup	3.5g	0.2g	0.1g	16
Mozzarella (whole milk)	1 oz.	0.6g	6.3g	6.3g	85
Mung bean	1/2	2g	1.5g	0g	16

Food	Serving Size	Net Carb	Protein	Fat	Calories
sprouts	cup				
Mushrooms, white	1/4 cup	1g	1g	0g	11
Mushrooms, shiitake	1/4 cup	4g	0.5g	0g	20
Mustard greens	1/2 cup	1.5g	2g	0.3g	18
Nopales (cactus pads)	1/2 cup	1g	1g	0g	11
Okra	1/2 cup	1.5g	1.5g	0g	18
Olive oil	1 Tbls	0g	0g	13.5g	119
Food	**Serving Size**	**Net Carb**	**Protein**	**Fat**	**Calories**
Olives, black	5	1g	0g	3g	30
Olives, green	5	0.1g	0g	2g	20

Onion, chopped	2 Tbls	1.5g	0.2g	0g	8
Parmesan	1 oz.	1g	10g	7.3g	111
Parsley	1 Tbls	0.1g	0.1g	0g	1
Pecans	10 halves	0.5g	1.3g	10g	98
Peppers, green bell	1/2 cup	2g	1g	0g	15
Peppers, green bell	1/4 cup	0.5g	0g	3.5g	37
Peppers, red bell	1/2 cup	3g	1g	0g	23
Peppers, red bell	1/4 cup	1.5g	0.3g	3.5g	35
Pine nuts	2 Tbls	0.7g	2.7g	14g	148
Pistachios	25 nuts	3g	3.5g	8g	98
Pumpkin	1/4	2g	0.5g	0g	12

Food	Serving Size	Net Carb	Protein	Fat	Calories
	cup				
Pumpkin seeds (hulled)	1/4 cup	1g	9g	14g	180
Radicchio	1/2 cup	0.8g	0.3g	0g	5
Radishes	6	0.2g	0g	0g	2
Food	**Serving Size**	**Net Carb**	**Protein**	**Fat**	**Calories**
Raspberries, fresh	1/4 cup	3.5g	0.4g	0.2g	16
Raspberries, frozen	1/4 cup	2g	0.4g	0.2g	18
Ricotta (whole milk)	1/2 cup	4g	14g	16g	216
Romaine lettuce	1 cup	0.5g	0.5g	0g	8
Sauerkraut	1/2 cup	1g	0.7g	0g	13

Scallion/green onion	1/4 cup	1g	0.5g	0g	8
Sesame seed oil	1 Tbls	0g	0g	13.6g	120
Sesame seeds	2 Tbls	2g	3.2g	9g	103
Shallots	2 Tbls	3g	0.5g	0g	14
Sour cream	1 Tbls	0.6g	0.3g	2.3g	24
Spaghetti squash	1/2 cup	4g	0.5g	0g	21
Spinach	1 cup	0.3g	1g	0g	7
Spinach	1/2 cup	1g	3g	0g	21
Strawberries, fresh, sliced	1/4 cup	2g	0.3g	0.2g	13
Strawberries, frozen	1/4 cup	2.5g	0.2g	0g	13
Strawberry, fresh	1 large	1g	0.1g	0.1g	6

Food	Serving Size	Net Carb	Protein	Fat	Calories
Summer squash	1/2 cup	2.5g	1g	0.4g	21
Sunflower seed butter	1 Tbls	3g	2.8g	9g	99
Sunflower seeds (hulled)	1/4 cup	3g	6g	15g	160
Swiss cheese	1 oz.	0.4g	7.6g	9g	111
Tahini (sesame paste)	1 Tbls	2g	2.6g	8g	89
Tomato	1 small	2.5g	1g	0g	16
Tomato	1/4 cup	2g	0.5g	0g	11
Tomato	1 medium	3.5g	1g	0.25g	22

Tomato, cherry	5	2.3g	1g	0.2g	15
Turnips	1/2 cup	3.5g	1g	0g	25
Walnut oil	1 Tbls	0g	0g	13.6	120
Walnuts	7 halves	1g	2g	9g	93
Watercress	1/2 cup	0.1g	0.4g	0g	2
Yogurt (plain unsweetened/whole milk)	1/2 cup	5.3	4g	3.7g	69
Zucchini	1/2 cup	1.5g	1g	0.3g	14

Spices and Sauces for Flavor

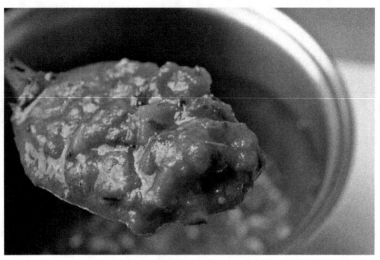

Because of the restrictions of the keto diet, sauces like ketchup and barbecue sauce have too much sugar and too many carbohydrates to include on your food list. Fortunately, most herbs have minimal amounts of carbohydrates. Spices have a little more carbs, but not so many that they are prohibited from the diet plan.

Here is a list of spices and herbs with nutritional information is based on 1teaspoon of herbs or spices.

NAME	NET CARBS	PROTEIN	FAT	CALORIES
Basil Leaves, Dried	2.21	1.09	0.19	11
Basil Leaves,	0.04	0.15	0.03	1.17

Fresh				
Bay Leaves, Dried	2.29	0.36	0.4	14.83
Black Pepper, Ground	1.82	0.49	0.15	11.83
Caraway Seed	0.56	0.93	0.69	15.67
Cardamom	1.92	0.51	0.32	14.67
Cayenne Pepper, Ground	1.39	0.57	0.82	15
Celery Flakes, Dried	1.69	0.53	0.1	15
Celery Seed	1.4	0.85	1.19	18.5
Chili Powder	0.7	0.64	0.68	13.33
Chives, Dried	1.81	1	0.17	14.67
Chives, Fresh	0.09	0.16	0.04	1.5
Cilantro, Dried	1.98	1.04	0.23	13.17
Cilantro, Fresh	0.04	0.1	0.03	1.17
Cinnamon, Ground	1.29	0.19	0.06	11.67

NAME	NET CARBS	PROTEIN	FAT	CALORIES
Clove, Ground	1.5	0.28	0.62	13
Coriander Seed	0.62	0.59	0.84	14
Coriander, Dried	1.98	1.04	0.23	13.17
Cumin Seed	1.59	0.84	1.05	17.67
Cumin, Ground	1.59	0.84	1.05	17.67
Curry Powder	0.12	0.68	0.66	15.33
Dill Weed, Dried	1.99	0.94	0.21	12
Dill Weed, Fresh	0.23	0.16	0.05	2
Fennel Seed	0.59	0.75	0.7	16.33
Garlic Powder	3	0.78	0.04	15.67
Ginger Root, Fresh	0.74	0.09	0.04	3.83
Ginger, Ground	2.72	0.43	0.2	15.83
Horseradish	0.21	0.03	0.02	1.21
Lemongrass,	1.2	0.09	0.02	4.67

NAME	NET CARBS	PROTEIN	FAT	CALORIES
Fresh				
Marjoram, Dried	0.96	0.6	0.33	12.83
Mustard, Ground	0.74	1.23	1.71	24
Nutmeg, Ground	1.35	0.28	1.72	24.83
Onion Powder	3.02	0.49	0.05	16.17
Oregano, Dried	1.26	0.43	0.2	12.5
Paprika, Ground	0.9	0.67	0.61	13.33
Parsley, Dried	1.13	1.26	0.26	13.83
Parsley, Fresh	0.015	0.14	0.04	1.67
Peppermint, Fresh	0.32	0.18	0.05	3.33
NAME	NET CARBS	PROTEIN	FAT	CALORIES
Poppy Seed	0.41	0.85	1.96	24.83
Red Pepper, Ground	1.39	0.57	0.82	15
Rosemary, Dried	1.01	0.23	0.72	15.67

Rosemary, Fresh	0.31	0.16	0.28	6.17
Saffron	2.91	0.54	0.28	14.67
Sage, Ground	0.97	0.5	0.6	14.83
Salt	0	0	0	0
Tarragon, Dried	2.02	1.08	0.34	14
Thyme, Dried	1.3	0.43	0.35	13
Thyme, Fresh	0.49	0.26	0.08	4.83
Turmeric Root	0.13	0.02	0.03	1.17
Turmeric, Ground	2.11	0.46	0.15	14.67
White Pepper, Ground	2.01	0.49	0.1	14

Since there are carbohydrates in most of the herbs and spices and calories as well, measure what you are adding to your food and count the amounts in your macros. The same is true for condiments. Below are the carb counts for low-carb condiments that fit into the keto diet.

FOOD	SERVING SIZE	NET CARBS (G)
Dressings, creamy (ranch, blue cheese, Caesar, etc.)	2 tbsp	2
Dressings, oil or vinaigrette	2 tbsp	2.7
Hot sauce (sriracha, buffalo, red pepper sauce, etc.)	1 tsp	1.2
FOOD	**SERVING SIZE**	**NET CARBS (G)**
Lemon juice, lime juice	2 tbsp	2.5
Marinara sauce	1/2 cup	7.4
Mayonnaise	1 tbsp	0.1
Mustard	1 tsp	0.1
Pesto sauce	1/4 cup	2.8
Salsa	2 tbsp	1.7
Vinegar – balsamic	1 tbsp	2.7
Vinegar – white, apple cider	1 tbsp	0

What Foods to Avoid

For the low carb portion of the diet, avoid grains, fruits with high sugar content, starchy vegetables, fruit juice and carrot juice, sugar (including honey and syrup), chips, crackers, and baked goods. These items are high in sugar and/or carbohydrates and will not be useful in a low-carbohydrate diet.

Fruits and Starchy Vegetables - Juice, fruit, and sugar are definite no-nos on the keto diet. The excess sugars will not only spike your carbohydrates, but they will also cause insulin to be released in response to the spike in blood sugar. This is all the opposite of the goal of ketosis. There will be too many carbohydrates available for the body to convert to energy. This will make it impossible for the body to be starved of carbs and glucose and the body will not switch to using fat as energy. Starchy vegetables like corn and beets have high sugar content. Bananas, apples, raisins, and mangoes are too high in sugar content to include on the keto diet. Fruit and sugar will have to be avoided to reach ketosis.

Grains, Bread, and Pasta - Grains are high in carbohydrates. Don't try to substitute grains with gluten-free bread and pasta. Even the gluten-free items tend to replace the grains with other foods that are also high in carbohydrates like chickpea flour. To replace pasta, try the zucchini spirals or shirataki noodles. These noodles are very low in carbohydrates and may be an alternative to high carb grain pasta that meets your needs. Butternut squash spirals are also readily available, but winter squash is high in carbohydrates. Quinoa is a protein-rich grain; there are too many carbohydrates for this grain to be included in the keto food list. Rice and potatoes, brown rice and sweet potatoes have too many carbs for even the healthy alternatives to be included in your food plan.

Legumes - Avoid beans and legumes like lentils, pinto, black beans, and chickpeas. Though they happen to be high in fiber, they unfortunately also are high in carbohydrates. That makes beans a poor addition to the ketogenic diet. They can be used sparingly when added in small amounts to recipes like soups and stews. They are nutritious, but like starchy vegetables, they do not fit well in the keto lifestyle.

Coated Meat -Meats with added sugar such as maple flavored sausage and bacon should be avoided. Also, breaded chicken and fish are not allowed on the keto diet. These foods have carbohydrates and are not options on the diet. It is better to eat food that is less processed, and if there are any added flavorings, you should add them yourself to maintain control of the additions.

Low Fat - Foods labeled as low fat often contain sugar or unapproved sugar substitutes, which act like sugar and trick your body into a spike in blood sugar and short term satisfaction. This is true for items you may not associate with sweet flavors like salad dressing and mayonnaise. In these instances, full-fat options are included on the keto diet so it's okay to eat the real food and avoid processed imitation.

Vegetable Oils - The nutritional value of vegetable, canola, and corn oils are not ideal for the keto diet. They like the nutritional values of higher quality oils and are high in polyunsaturated fatty acids (PUFA). These PUFAs are bad for your heart as they release plaque into arteries. They also cause inflammation in the liver and may promote liver disease. In fact, vegetable oils may be a cause of obesity. Vegetable oil is unhealthy.

Of course, most foods are technically allowed on the ketogenic diet. In order to include some of these forbidden foods in your diet and remain in ketosis, measure your foods and flavorings and know what you are consuming when it comes to carbohydrates and overall calories. Because the consumption of carbohydrates spikes blood sugar levels, when blood sugar drops, there will be a feeling of malaise and hunger when the carbohydrates wear off. It is better to eat more calories from foods that will sustain a constant level of blood sugar and foods that will help keep your stomach feeling full.

Keto Approved Sweeteners

On this very low carb diet, sugar and sweetener are eliminated. There is no room in the diet for sugar-based carbohydrates. Fortunately, there are substitutes that can be used in place of sugar if you are baking keto items or even to add to coffee or tea. The best sweeteners on keto are stevia and erythritol. These can be used independently or combined.

There are several sweeteners that are keto-friendly:

Sweetener	Measure	Type	Net Carbs	Calories
Stevia	1/2 Cup	Natural	5	20
Monk Fruit	1/2 Cup	Natural	25	100
Erythritol	1/2 Cup	Sugar Alcohol	5	20
Sucralose	1/2 Cup	Artificial	0	0
Aspartame	1/2 Cup	Artificial	85	352
Saccharin	1/2 Cup	Artificial	94	364
Table Sugar	1/2 Cup	Processed	100	387

Stevia and erythritol are both plant-based sweeteners that can be used in place of sugar and but with drastically fewer calories. Stevia three times sweeter than sugar, erythritol is nearly twice as sweet as sugar. Because they are sweeter than sugar, it is not necessary to use as much of the sweeteners are you would use sugar. Stevia is a plant, the leaves of which are naturally sweet. Stevia is available in powder form, granulated and liquid form.

Erythritol is derived from plants, as well. The plants must be processed and the sweetness is extracted through a fermentation of plant leaves when sugar alcohols are extracted. The resulting sugar alcohol can be up to 80% sweeter than regular sugar. Erythritol is only available in granulated form. Erythritol is not absorbed completely by the body. This is one of the reasons it fits into the keto diet. Because it is not completely absorbed, it does not greatly affect insulin production.

Both stevia and erythritol can be used in baking on a keto diet. The two artificial sweeteners do not melt as quickly as regular sugar, so there may be some modifications necessary for successful baking. Since they are both commercially prepared, it may be that additives affect the number of carbs in the finished product in an effort to produce a consistent product.

Keto on a Budget

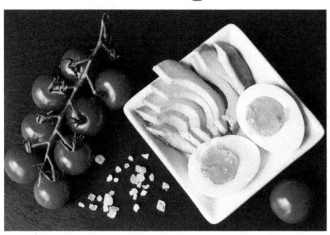

One of the things that people say against the keto diet is that it is expensive. In reality, it doesn't have to be expensive. You can do the keto diet for the same amount of money as any other food plan. The recommendations for grass-fed beef and organic produce are recommendations. It's true that grass-fed beef is healthier. But you will be able to reach ketosis without grass-fed meat. Some of the items are more expensive, that is just a fact. But you are investing in yourself, and you are worth it. While you may be spending more money on your food that you're purchasing, you will also be saving money on food that you previously purchased but no longer suits your lifestyle. There will be no more sugary snacks, no more potato chips. These items cost a lot of money as well. By eating fresh foods, you will be saving yourself money.

So, if you're on a budget doing keto, the first thing you should do is to try to locate items on the diet at a lower cost.

Be sure to see what you can find on the internet. Look for items in retail stores in your area that you know are less expensive than other stores. Organic products and grass-fed meats are available in most communities. They are more expensive, but you may be able to find them at a lower price at different locations. This is especially true if you seek out some of the items on the internet.

Though organic products are easy to find, one of the main advantages of the keto diet is that its not necessary to eat organic produce, and you don't have to ingest grass-fed meats. You do want to get the best quality that you can. When you're addressing your diet, you may just be moving your food dollars from one category of food to another category of food. In other words, some foods that you are used to buying may fall off your list entirely. Also, it is not necessary to purchase prepackaged ketogenic foods. These products are manufactured for a variety of diets, and many times, they just put a keto-friendly label on the box to sell it. These foods may contain more carbohydrates than you want to consume. Remember, there are several kinds of keto diets. What may work on one keto diet may not work for your keto diet. Besides, since you will be preparing many meals, you can add snack bars and snack foods to your ketogenic baking repertoire. The keto snacks are typically expensive. By making the snacks yourself, you will be saving money and controlling what nutrients you include in your diet.

You can use your food dollars to be creative with food, and if you are accustomed to not preparing your own food, you may find that you're saving money in the long run by not consistently eating out. Just like any other budget item, there is usually a way to work around restrictions of your budget. You can be on the keto diet without breaking your budget by purchasing items in bulk like nuts and flours. The internet offers a lot of opportunities to save money while you're on the keto diet. Stay away from processed foods even keto-friendly foods. It is very possible to be on the ketogenic diet without spending more money. When you eliminate processed foods from your budget, you end up with fresh foods and you control your intake of those foods. It may be necessary to plan a menu and use your menu to determine your grocery list. In the end, you may end up saving money because you only purchase what is on your list and staples for your pantry. You may find that you are not spending more money even if you purchase grass-fed meats and organic products. This is because impulse buys are eliminated and you stick to what you need and do not purchase items that are extraneous to your budget.

Keto Away From Home

The ketogenic diet needs to travel with you no matter where you are. At times you may need to go to parties or may want to go to parties and gatherings, and you may fear the temptations of food items at the party. One way to eliminate the worry is to prepare something and take it with you to the party. If you bring an item for everyone to enjoy, you will be providing a hostess gift as well as a dish that you know you can eat. That way you will not be stuck eating crudités and drinking water. You will be able to prepare an item that you enjoy and that others will enjoy with you.

If you are friendly with the host or hostess of the party, you may be able to ascertain what they're serving at the party and know whether you can indulge in items at the gathering. Especially as we get older, we realize that more and more people have dietary restrictions. It is not uncommon for people to have restrictions and for hosts of parties to prepare for the restrictions of others. In society today, there are many people who are gluten-free, carb-free or have other food allergies. As a result, people are accustomed to preparing foods or having food available that people with such restrictions may eat while at the gatherings. So if you have a relationship with the host, you may be able to determine what they're serving and if you can bring something that suits your dietary needs as well as that of others.

If you are not in a position to be able to ask what is being served, and you don't feel comfortable bringing something of your own, it's a good idea to eat prior to leaving the house. That way, you will not feel like you must indulge due to hunger and you will be in a better frame of mind to pick and choose from the food offered. There is usually something that you will be able to eat at a party, even if it is not fulfilling. If you have eaten prior to leaving that you're home, you will not be ravenous and you can partake in the items that you are able to eat and leave the items that are not on your diet on the platter. If these gatherings involve alcohol, the keto diet only allows for the consumption of dry wines and hard spirits. If you are drinking hard liquor, use water or club soda as a mixer. Tonic water has carbohydrates in it and is not appropriate on the keto diet.

Keto at Restaurants

Eating in restaurants is not as difficult as eating in someone's home. Because of the sustained and massive interest in the ketogenic diet and other diets of its kind, there are many restaurants that offer low-carbohydrate versions of meals. At fast-food restaurants, typically you would simply order a burger or grilled chicken without the bun without ketchup or barbeque sauce Use lettuce as your bun. Of course, you will pass on the fries and onion rings. In general, fast food dining will not be your best option for eating out on a keto diet.

Restaurants with more items available, like sit-down restaurants, have larger menus and the choices often include many items that you can order or have modified and follow the ketogenic plan. The biggest problem you will have at these restaurants is the portion size. You need to be aware that the huge portion sizes are not going to be conducive to your eating plan. Remember to stay within your calories for the day. If you order food at a restaurant you will typically get enough food for two people. For this reason, you may want to split an entree with someone else who is dining with you. Also, if there are items on the menu with your entree that are not on the keto diet, request to have them left off your plate. This will save the kitchen waste and save you the temptation of eating items that are not on your diet plan. Many restaurants have their menu on the internet. It is a good idea to review the selections and have an idea of what you want to order when you get to the restaurant. Order two vegetables for sides of the entrees. Make sure the vegetables are ketogenic friendly. Stay away from the potatoes and the rice. You can generally order two vegetables. If you're not able to order to split an order, make sure you divide your order in half before you begin eating. Some people like to order the carryout container to be delivered with their food. This way they move half of their portion into the container before they start to eat. This is a good idea if you feel like you will not be able to stop eating once you start.

The keto diet is easy to follow in most restaurants in situations, but the portions are large and you should make sure you do not overeat and do not exceed your calorie counts nor other macros for in your restaurant meal.

Chapter 4: What are the Best Fats on Keto?

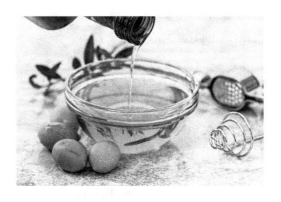

Fats are the most important part of the keto diet, but which fats are best for the diet? There are a variety of fats that can be used. The fat eaten on the keto diet makes up 70% of the food that you'll be eating each day. This makes the types of fats eaten important because all fats are not going to produce healthy weight loss on the keto diet. There are fats to be consumed and fats to be avoided. Just because fat is the predominant macro does that mean that consumption of unlimited fat is part of the keto diet. Stay within your calorie allotment for the day and watch your macros. Do not exceed your macros when you're eating fats. Most importantly, consume the correct types of fat to maximize the effectiveness of your fat intake.

Types of Fat

There are several types of fat and some are better than others when it comes to overall health and usefulness as fuel for the body. Combine various types of fats that have proved to be the best fuel for the body.

Polyunsaturated Fatty Acids (PUFA)

These are fats with some health contributions but not as many as other unsaturated and saturated fats. This is the category where omega-3 fatty acids fall. Omega-3 fatty acids are good for the brain and should be included in a healthy diet. The problems with PFUAs arise when they are heated because they may, with heat, form compounds that cause inflammation, and I may damage the pancreas and liver.

Polyunsaturated fatty acids (PFUA) should be eaten cold to avoid the unstable reactions of PUFAs when heated. Some good PFUAs for the keto diet are extra virgin olive oil, nuts, avocados and avocado oil, and fatty fish.

Monounsaturated Fatty Acids (MUFAs)

These fats are the healthiest of unsaturated fats. They remain stable when heated and have a positive effect on insulin production and cholesterol levels. MUFAs assist the pancreas in producing and consistent levels of insulin. They are also known to reduce bad cholesterol levels (LDL) and improve overall blood pressure and heart health.

The MUFAs are commonly found in lard, bacon, macadamia nuts, sesame oil, and butter. These fats remain stable at higher temperatures and therefore have predictable reactions to heat. These oils can be moderately included in the keto diet.

Saturated Fats

These are the best fats for keto. They are found in animals, and other high-fat foods and are not the result of chemical processing. When eating fats on keto, hunger is assuaged by the consumption of saturated fats. These fats have a positive influence on the health of the body. Included in saturated fats is MCT oil. MCT stands for Medium Chain Triglycerides. The shorter length of triglyceride makes MCTs easier to digest and break down in the system. MCTs are known to improve brain function and reduce the growth of yeast and bacteria in the body. It's a beneficial oil while on keto.

Saturated fats are known to increase the amount of good cholesterol, HDL while decreasing the bad cholesterol, LDL. There is also an improvement to the immune system and an increase in bone density when saturated fats are present in the human body. This is a good side effect for women over 50 who may be suffering from bone loss.

Common foods that are good sources of healthy saturated fats are fatty meats like steak, butter and ghee, eggs, coconut oil, lard, and palm kernel oil. These items should be included in the majority of fat on the keto diet. Since the diet relies on the consumption of so much fat, there will be a need to eat a lot of these fats. This will be the healthiest way to provide fat as fuel for your body as you reduce the number of carbs in your diet.

Omega-3, Omega-6, Omega-9

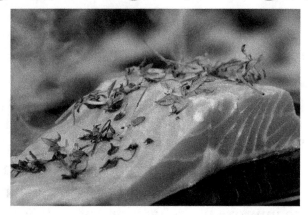

Omega-3 fatty acids are polyunsaturated fats that increase HDL and improve heart health. They decrease the fat in the liver and improve liver function. These fats also reduce the inflammation in your body and organs. Omega-3 fatty acids are key in reducing waist size and promoting weight loss. Foods high in omega-3 fatty acids are fish, like salmon, mackerel, and sardines. Walnuts and chia seeds are also high in Omega-3.

Omega-6 fatty acids are polyunsaturated fats that are used for energy. The problem is, most normal diets contain too much Omega-6. In large concentrations, the omega-6 fatty acids increase inflammation in the body and cause associated diseases like asthma, rheumatoid arthritis, ulcerative colitis, and sinusitis. Omega-6 fatty acids must be consumed in moderation so that negative effects do not overwhelm the positive. Some of the foods high in omega-6 are soybean oil, corn oil, mayonnaise, walnuts, and almonds. Eating these foods in moderation will be the best way to receive the benefits of omega-6 fatty acids.

Omega-9 fatty acids are monounsaturated fats that are found naturally in the body but may be consumed as well. These fats are found to improve the worst types of cholesterol in the body, reduce inflammation and improve insulin sensitivity. They may also improve metabolism when monounsaturated fats with omega-9 are consumed instead of saturated fats. Foods high in omega-9 are nut and seed oils like cashew oil, flaxseed oil, peanut oil, and olive oil. It is also found in olives as well as almonds, cashews, and walnuts. Moderate consumption of omega-9 fatty acids is appropriate because it is a natural part of the body's composition and tolerated well when introduced as food.

Fats play an important role in the keto diet. Foods with Omega-3 fatty acids should get added to your food plan two or three times a week. Omega-6 fatty acids should not be included in a grand way in the diet as they do not have as many positive effects on the body. Overconsumption of omega-6 can have negative effects on overall health. Omega-9 fatty acids are already found in the body so it isn't necessary to work hard getting it into your system.

Fat Bombs

With all the talk about fats, let's not overlook fat bombs. Fat bombs are high-fat morsels of food used to boost fat levels while on the keto diet. This is good if you find that you are not eating enough fat or feel hungry or lacking in energy. These items are high in fat, low in carbohydrates and combined into a small portion designed to boost energy, reduces cravings and fill you up so you don't feel hungry. Because of the small size, do not overindulge. They are meant to be small bites that last. Pay attention to your macros, even while indulging in little bursts of food energy.

Chapter 5: Negative Moments in Keto

Keto Flu

Keto flu is the feeling of fatigue, headache, and the lack of concentration similar to being sick with the flu. It occurs when eliminating carbohydrates from the system. The body is adjusting to the lack of carbohydrates by offering a barrage of warnings that something is missing. Eventually, the transition will be complete and energy will be derived from fat instead of carbohydrates, but how to get through the keto flu?

If possible, avoid the keto flu. To do this, gradually reduce the carbohydrates and your system, so your body is able to adapt from the primary energy source of carbohydrates to the new source of fat. Eliminate processed carbohydrates from your diet first. These carbohydrates are sugar, cereals, baked goods, and packaged items with preservatives and salt. Eliminating these foods will give a good start to avoiding the keto flu. It is good to kick off your quest for ketosis by getting rid of it the least healthy foods first. Next, stop eating grains. For many people, this is a difficult category of food to stop eating. The carbohydrates in bread, rice, wheat flour, and pasta provide a lot of energy in a regular diet. People consider many of these carbohydrates to be comfort food. It is hard to give them up. Fortunately, your body can adjust to being without them. Finally, eliminate fruits and starchy vegetables. Weaning yourself off carbs is a way to reduce the effects of withdrawal on the body as the fuel stores of carbohydrates and glucose are used up and ketosis takes over and your body begins getting energy from fat.

When you are reducing the number of carbohydrates, be sure to drink a lot of water. The reduction of carbohydrates will, from the start, release the water stored in your body and increase the frequency of urination. When you stay hydrated, that removes an unnecessary stressor from your system as you adjust to the reduction of carbohydrates. Also, replace electrolytes being removed with your frequent trips to the bathroom. Replenish them with high potassium, low carbohydrate foods like salmon, nuts, mushrooms, and green leafy vegetables. Trying to keep electrolytes in balance and avoid the keto flu. You may also supplement your hydration with bone broth. Heat the bone broth and add salt and seasonings this will help restore your electrolyte balance as well.

If you're unable to avoid the keto flu, you want to feel better fast. One of the best ways to manage the effects of keto flu is to drink lots of water and get lots of sleep. These two things reduce the amount of stress your body is feeling and allowed to switch the generation energy from carbohydrates def bad which will mean you're finally in ketosis. Stay the course and stick to the diet. The keto flu symptoms will eventually pass. If you and the bone broth to your diet while you're feeling the effects of the keto flu, it will provide essential nutrients and comfort from the warm of the beverage in your stomach. iI essence, you are treating the keto flu in the same way you would treat regular flu. Allow your body to rest and drink lots of water but stay the course on your diet so that you reach ketosis which will end your keto flu.

Constipation

You may find that as you eliminate grains from your diet, your bowel movements are not your friend. Your body should be able to adjust to the change in food over time but you may need to introduce foods that will promote easy evacuation. Doctors have said that difficulty in bowel movements is uncomfortable but not usually a serious ailment. You will probably be able to last for some time with the mental challenge of straining to poop, but you don't really want to endure the pain, so make sure you incorporate whole fiber whole grains into your diet so that you are able to move your bowels. Some suggestions are to add chia seeds and flax seeds to your diet in order to lessen the effects of constipation. Add chia seeds to water, stir and drink. The chia seeds don't have any flavor and even the pickiest eaters should be able to stomach the watery concoction. One or two tablespoons of chia seeds may be just what you need to relieve yourself of constipation. If you add the chia seeds to yogurt or smoothies, you run the risk of exceeding your carbohydrate macros. The problem with this yogurt and dairy tends to be high in carbohydrates so you may end up using your daily allotment of carbohydrates on one food item.

Diarrhea

On the other side of constipation is diarrhea. If you're experiencing diarrhea on the keto diet, it may be as simple as your consuming too much fat and too much protein. When the fat and protein are not digested easily, they're not absorbed into your system and remain unused and diarrhea is the result. Consume more fiber and look at the fat you're eating. If you are not meeting your macros, make an effort to fix them. Try changing over to monounsaturated fats and MCTs that are easily absorbed into the body and that may be able to fix your problem with diarrhea. Brussel sprouts, avocado, and broccoli are keto-friendly soluble fibers that will help with constipation.

Dietary changes may upset your system and may show itself in a negative way through constipation or diarrhea and upset stomach. It's good to make notes of what you are eating and compare it to your macros to be sure that your every sure you're eating good fat and that some of your protein comes from some of your protein is coming from vegetable green leafy vegetables. Adding a whole grain may help, as well.

Insomnia

An inability to sleep may accompany your keto diet. Energy from carbohydrates is not sustained over long periods of time. As the carbohydrates are leaving the body, it may be that the body is not dependent on carbohydrates and does not experience the crash when the carbs are used up. It is usually a temporary condition,

To combat sleeplessness, try a few different things:

1. Eat your carbohydrates closer to bedtime. This may trick your body into a state of low energy in a simulation of what often happens when you get your energy from carbohydrates. Just as you have a burst of energy upon eating carbs, the energy is quickly dissipated, and a feeling of tiredness and lethargy ensues.
2. Replenish electrolytes in your body through potassium-rich foods that will provide essential nutrients to your body, which may be missing and through your body out of balance. Avocados, pumpkin seeds, and salmon are helpful foods in counteracting the loss of minerals.
3. Prepare for bed. Make sure the room is dark and comfortable, and consider meditation or yoga before bedtime.

Diet Plateaus

When you have been losing weight, and it suddenly stops, it can be an irritating situation. Plateaus are common in all diets. The body adjusts to what you are eating and what you are doing for exercise and settles in. To get through the plateau, a change will need to be made.

The first thing to do if your weight loss is slower than expected is to review your macros. Every four or five weeks, you should recalculate your macros to make adjustments for your weight loss. A plateau may be the result of overeating your macros. Be sure you are not exceeding your overall daily calorie count. If your calories are not all burned off with activity, you will not lose weight. Your calories expended must exceed calories eaten to lose weight. Keep track of everything you eat, even little things, and include them in your macros. It will help you know you are not exceeding overall calories.

If you are not exercising, exercise. If you are exercising, you may need to change your routine. Increased exercise will jolt the body into a new use of energy and be forced to burn more energy, and as a result, more fat. It isn't about where you are exercising or that you are in the gym or jogging; you may just need to add steps to your day or increase your activity. You just need to increase your movement.

If your macros are still accurate and you are not losing weight, consider measuring yourself on a regular basis, especially if you have added exercise and weight training to our daily routine. Muscle weighs more than fat, be sure you are not replacing fat with muscle. That is not a bad situation to be in, but you should know if you are actually doing well, and your body is gaining strength and muscle. If you have not adjusted your workout routine, this probably isn't the problem.

Other things that may cause weight gain are stress and sleeplessness, which causes stress in the body. Stress is something that causes the body to retain weight as it gears up to fight whatever it is that is causing the turmoil in your body. Exercise may help to relieve stress. So will meditation or yoga. The key is to relieve yourself of the stress so your body may be more efficiently working on your weight loss.

Cholesterol and Keto

There are many food staples of the keto diet that are known to increase cholesterol levels in humans. This is one of the reasons food quality is part of the diet plan. For some of the food items on the plan, the higher quality items have fewer negative effects on healthy eating.

Cholesterol is a type of fat in your blood. It is formed in the liver and distributed throughout the body through the arteries and veins. Cholesterol, in normal amounts, travels to the brain and helps the brain function and memory. It also helps in the generation of hormones and normal organ functions, including the largest organ, skin. If there is too much cholesterol in the blood, the fats cling to the walls of the veins and arteries and may cause clogs or restrict the flow of blood. When there is not enough blood moving to the heart, a heart attack may result. If there is not enough blood reaching the brain, a stroke may occur. This is why the level of cholesterol in the system is a key factor in determining the health of an individual.

Cholesterol is made up of two types of lipoprotein. There is low-density lipoprotein (LDL), which moves through the blood with the assistance of proteins and other substances in the blood that causes plaque. Plaque is what attaches the fat to the walls of the veins. This is why LDL is considered to be bad cholesterol. High-density lipoprotein (HDL) is healthy cholesterol. It does not accumulate as it moves through the bloodstream. It carries cholesterol with it as it moves through blood vessels and takes it to the liver where it is processed for evacuation from the body.

Since the keto diet is one that concentrates on consuming so much fat, choosing appropriate fats will give you some control over the type of cholesterol in your body. The body needs cholesterol to function properly, so the goal is to consume food products prone to add more HDL and minimal amounts of LDL to your blood. To do this, the fats you eat should not have trans fats. Trans fats are high in LDL. They are often found in packaged foods, fried foods, margarine, baked goods, and crackers. Well, most of these items are not part of the keto diet. When prepared with partially or hydrogenated cooking oils, even fried meats are subject to higher levels of LDL. They are often used because they are more stable at higher temperatures.

If you are eating the right fats and find that your cholesterol levels are being negatively affected by the keto diet, try changing what you are eating as well as the combinations of food. If you are following the gentle keto 10% carb diet try reducing the number of carbs in your diet. Studies have found that people on a low-carb diet have increased HDL levels while they are losing weight. You may also try to limit your oils consumed to extra virgin olive oil which has been found to increase HDL as it is less processed than some other oils. Increased exercise is a way to combat low levels of HDL. Exercise will help you lose more weight as well. Losing weight helps with cholesterol levels.

For most people, the keto diet will not adversely affect cholesterol levels and, in fact, may improve the ratios between HDL and LDL levels. If you have cholesterol concerns, check with your doctor to be sure it is monitored regularly. Each body is different, and so you may have to try different methods of controlling your cholesterol levels. With the help of your physician, you should be able to determine if changes are working. A lower weight may be the best improvement to your health.

Chapter 6: Keto Recipes

Breakfast

Keto-Friendly Breakfast Tortilla

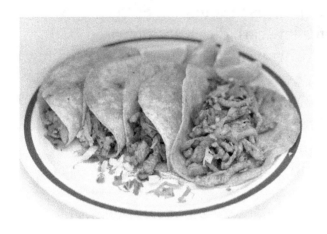

This breakfast tortilla recipe is replacing a flour burrito with an eggy wrap. This can be used to make an easy hand-held breakfast omelet for a compact keto breakfast.

Prep & Cooking Time: 10 mins

Servings: 1 tortilla
Nutrition Facts: Calories: 331 | Carbohydrates: 1g | Protein: 11g | Fat: 30g
Ingredients

1 T. butter

2 large eggs
2 T cream cheese
1 t. chilli powder
salt to taste

Instructions:

1. Melt cream cheese in a microwave for 10 seconds at a time until soft. Whisk until smooth.
2. Mix in eggs, chili powder, and salt.
3. Melt butter in a pan on medium heat. When melted, pour egg mixture in a pan and spread around in a circle. To thinly and evenly coat the bottom of the pan.
4. Turn the heat to low and cover the pan, so the top of the egg mixture cooks.
5. Leave on heat until the top of the egg mixture is dry- around 2 minutes.
6. Slide out egg onto the pan onto a plate.
7. Fill the keto tortilla with your choice of meat, cheese, and vegetables.
8. Roll up the "tortilla" and eat immediately or let cool and wrap in paper to enjoy later.

Breakfast Sandwich

You don't need bread when you can use sausage instead. The sausage patties are easy to handle and prove the perfect accompaniment to the eggs and cheese for with plenty of fat to start your keto day. This is perfect as a 'breakfast for dinner' meal if you add a vegetable like spinach or baby kale instead of avocado.

Prep & Cooking Time: 15 mins

Servings: 1 sandwich
Nutrition Facts: Calories: 603 | Carbohydrates: 7g | Protein: 22g | Fat: 54g

Ingredients:

2 pork sausage patties
1 large egg
1 T cream cheese
2 T sharp cheddar or extra sharp cheddar cheese

¼ medium avocado, sliced

Sriracha to taste
Salt and pepper to taste

Instructions

1. Cook sausages in a skillet over medium heat until the sausage is cooked through. Do this according to the package instructions.
2. Place the cream cheese and cheddar cheese in a microwave-safe bowl. Heat the cheeses until melted. This will take 20 or 30 seconds depending on your microwave.
3. Add sriracha to the cheese to taste and set the bowl aside.
4. Beat eggs in a different bowl and add salt and pepper as desired.
5. Coat frying pan with oil and butter. Cook egg as omelet until done.
6. Add avocado to egg, fold, and remove from pan.
7. Spread both sausage patties with cream cheese mixture.
8. Assemble the sandwich by layering sausage, egg, and top with a sausage patty.
9. Serve while hot.

Banana Nut Muffins

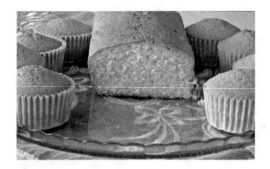

That's right; banana muffins are keto. Just use banana extract instead of bananas to get that familiar flavor. The muffin makes a great nut-holder as well. This is keto baking at its finest.

Prep & Cooking Time: 45 mins

Servings: 1 muffin
Nutrition Facts: Calories: 184 | Carbohydrates: 7g | Protein: 7g | Fat: 14g

Ingredients:

1 ¼ c almond flour
¼ c stevia
2 t baking powder
½ t ground cinnamon
⅓ c butter, melted
2 ½ t banana extract

¼ c unsweetened vanilla almond milk

¼ c sour cream
2 large eggs, slightly beaten
¾ c finely chopped walnuts or pecans

Topping:

1 T cold butter cut into pieces

1 T almond flour
½ T stevia

Instructions:

Preheat oven to 350 degrees
Grease a muffin tin with butter or line with 10 muffin liners.

Mix muffins

1. In a large bowl, mix dry ingredients, including the cinnamon.
2. Stir in melted butter, banana extract, almond milk, and sour cream.
3. Add eggs and nuts to the mixture and mix until all ingredients are incorporated.
4. Fill muffin cups with batter to half full.

Crumble topping:

1. Pulse the cold butter, almond flour, and stevia in a food processor until crumbly. If the mixture appears too dry, add another tablespoon of butter to pulse a few more times.
2. Sprinkle topping on top of muffins evenly.

Bake: 20 minutes.

Remove from oven when golden brown and they appear cooked. Let cool before eating. The texture will not be the same as a muffin but denser. They are still tasty little bites for breakfast.

Smoothies and Beverages

Coconut Green Smoothie

This smoothie has coconut oil and coconut milk as a wonderful pick-me-up when you need a shot of fiber. Enjoy the fresh coconut flavor that is balanced with matcha. It is a refreshing drink for any time.

Prep Time: 5 mins

Servings: 1 smoothie
Nutrition Facts: Calories: 341 | Carbohydrates: 3.9g | Protein: 5.6g | Fat: 24.7g

Ingredients:
⅔ c slightly defrosted frozen chopped spinach
½ avocado
1 T coconut oil
½ t matcha powder
1 T monk fruit sweetener
½ c coconut milk (from the dairy section, not canned)
⅔ c water
½ cup of ice

Instructions:

1. Add all ingredients except the ice into a blender. Blend until everything is blended well.
2. Pulse in the ice until it is evenly distributed.

3. Pour into a glass.

This smoothie is good for fiber and fat. You can add flaxseed or softened chia seeds to the smoothie for additional fiber and nutrients. Fresh spinach can be used and may be substituted with fresh or frozen kale.

Strawberry Smoothie

Add a touch of sweetness to your day with this strawberry smoothie. This smoothie is good enough for dessert. If you want to add some fiber and protein, try adding chia seeds that have been softened in water. 2 tablespoons of chia will add 139 calories, 1 gram of carbohydrate, 4 grams of protein, and 9 grams of fat.

Prep Time: 5 mins

Servings: 1 smoothie
Nutrition Facts: Calories: 302 | Carbohydrates: 8g | Protein: 2g | Fat: 26g

Ingredients:

¼ c heavy cream
¾ c unsweetened vanilla almond milk
2 t stevia
½ c frozen strawberries (whole or sliced)
½ c ice (preferably crushed)

Instructions:

1. Blend ingredients in a blender until blended well.
2. Pour into a tall glass.
3. Serve.

Keto Mojito

Yes! There are keto-friendly cocktails. It takes a little preparation; stevia is used instead of sugar, but you don't need a blender. Muddling the mint leaves releases the mint fragrance and provides the minty backdrop for this refreshing drink. This is an easy recipe that is festive and interactive (muddling) for a fun part beverage.

Prep Time: 4 mins

Servings: 1 mojito
Nutrition Facts: Calories: 109 | Carbohydrates: 2g

Ingredients
4 fresh mint leaves
2 T fresh lime Juice
2 t stevia
Ice
1.5 oz shot of white rum

splash club soda or plain seltzer
fresh mint as garnish

Instructions:

1. Muddle the mint, lime juice, and stevia for 10 seconds in the glass in which the drink will be served.
2. Fill the glass with ice, either cubed or crushed.
3. Pour the shot of vodka over the ice.
4. Add club soda to fill the glass
5. Garnish with a mint leaf.

You may want to strain the drink after muddling to remove the broken mint leaves, so they don't get in the way of enjoying the drink. You can substitute vodka or gin for rum.

Soup

Chicken and Riced Cauliflower Soup

To make this soup keto-friendly, riced cauliflower is used to add that missing texture to the soup. It is a hearty soup that will remind you of homemade soups from home...or the deli. It makes a nice lunch or snack. Make a batch on the weekend and take it for lunch through the week.

Prep & Cooking Time: 40 mins

Servings: 4 Servings
Nutrition Facts: Calories: 196 | Carbohydrates: 4.8g | Protein: 26.4g | Fat: 10.4g

Ingredients:

2 T olive oil
2 stalks celery with tops, chopped
¼ c onions, chopped
salt and pepper, to taste
2 cloves garlic, minced
½ t paprika
4 c unsalted organic chicken bone broth
2 c chicken thigh meat, cut into 1/2" cubes
2 c riced cauliflower

Instructions:
1. Heat the oil in a large saucepan over medium heat.

2. Add celery and onions and season with salt and pepper. Cook, stirring frequently, until vegetables are tender, about 5 minutes.
3. Add garlic and paprika. If needed, add another tablespoon of olive oil to the pan with the garlic, so the garlic cooks evenly. Saute and cook until garlic is soft. This will take a minute or so.
4. Stir in chicken bone broth and bring to a boil.
5. Add chicken and riced cauliflower and simmer the soup until the chicken is cooked and the cauliflower is tender, but not overcooked.
6. Season with additional salt and pepper to taste.
7. Serve hot.

Spicy Creamy Chicken Soup

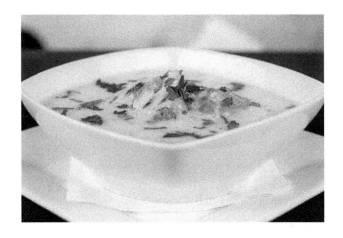

This recipe uses a slow-cooker to make soup in one pot. It is a spicy soup that has a lot of flavors and is high in fat. The heat of the jalapeño is offset by the cream cheeses. The soup tastes like a taco dip with chicken. Use the bone in chicken breasts to keep the chicken from drying out for the slow cook on low heat.

Prep & Cooking Time: 4 hrs 20 mins

Servings: 4 Servings
Nutrition Facts: Calories: 424 | Carbohydrates: 6g | Protein: 41g | Fat: 25g

Ingredients:

1 lb chicken breasts on the bone
1 c onion, diced
4 cloves garlic, minced
1 jalapeño pepper, chopped
1 T cumin
½ T chili powder
1 t salt
3 T lime juice
2 c low sodium organic chicken broth
1 8 oz package of cream cheese
½ c cilantro, chopped

Instructions:

1. Add the chicken, onion, garlic, jalapeño, cumin, chili powder, paprika, salt, lime juice, and chicken broth to a slow cooker.
2. Cook in the slow-cooker, covered, for 4 hours on the lowest setting.
3. After chicken is cooked through, remove from the pot and let cool until it can be easily handled.
4. Pull the chicken off the bone and shred or chop into bite-sized pieces.
5. Add the cream cheese to hot soup. Stir slowly until melted.
6. Add shredded chicken into the pot and stir to mix.
7. Bring the soup back up to temperature and turn off the heat.

8. Spoon into bowls and sprinkle cilantro on top.
9. Serve immediately.

Add a sprinkle of cheddar to add cheesy flavor to the soup.

Broccoli Cheese Soup

This is a thick and hearty soup that only has 5 ingredients. This can serve as a quick, last-minute meal that will please everyone. If you want to make it even more hearty, add tender cooked cubes of beef.

Prep & Cooking Time: 45 mins

Servings: 6 Servings
Nutrition Facts: Calories: 291 | Carbohydrates: 4g | Protein: 13g | Fat: 25g

Ingredients:

4 c broccoli florets
4 cloves minced garlic
3 ½ c low sodium vegetable broth
1 c heavy cream
3 c shredded sharp cheddar cheese

INSTRUCTIONS

1. In a large pot, sauté garlic in butter, ghee, or olive oil for one minute over medium heat.

2. Add vegetable broth, heavy cream, and chopped broccoli.
3. Heat soup to boiling, then reduce heat and simmer for 10-20 minutes, until broccoli is tender.
4. Use an immersion blender to puree the broccoli in the soup. If you do not have an immersion blender, use a slotted spoon to remove the broccoli and blend in a blender or food processor. After the broccoli is pureed, stir it back into the soup pot.
5. Reduce the heat under the soup and slowly add the cheddar into the soup, stirring frequently until melted.
6. Puree the soup again with the stick blender or regular blender.
7. Remove the soup from heat and serve in bowls.

Sauces and Dips

Tzatziki

Tzatziki can be used as a sauce or topping or dip. It is so versatile; add it to a salad of lettuce, tomato, olives, and arugula. It can be a dip for meat skewers or a spread for a keto-friendly sandwich. Tzatziki is a fresh, light addition to any snack or meal.

Prep Time: 10 mins

Servings: 8 Servings, 2 tablespoons per serving
Nutrition Facts: Calories: 79 | Carbohydrates: 3g | Protein: 1g | Fat: 7g

Ingredients:

½ c shredded cucumber, drained
1 tsp salt
1 T olive oil
1 T fresh mint, finely chopped
2 garlic cloves
1 c full-fat Greek yogurt
1 t lemon juice

Instructions:

1. Place shredded cucumber on a strainer for an hour or squeeze out moisture through a cheesecloth.

2. Mix all ingredients in a medium bowl
3. Refrigerate.

Use as a vegetable dip, a dip for dehydrated vegetables, or a sauce for lamb, beef, or chicken. It is also a perfect accompaniment for fried summer squash.

Satay Sauce

Bring a bit of Thailand into your kitchen with this satay sauce recipe. This is a great use for peanut butter and coconut cream. It is simply delicious and naturally keto-friendly.

Prep & Cooking Time: 15 mins

Servings: 4 Servings
Nutrition Facts: Calories: 312 | Carbohydrates: 7g | Protein: 7g | Fat: 30g

Ingredients:
1 can (14 oz) coconut cream (if you can't find coconut cream, coconut milk works well)
1 dry red pepper, seeds removed, chopped fine
1 clove garlic, minced
¼ c gluten-free soy sauce
⅓ c natural unsweetened peanut butter
salt and pepper

Instructions:

1. Place all ingredients in a small saucepan.
2. Bring the mixture to a boil
3. Stir while heating to mix peanut butter with other ingredients as it melts.
4. After the mixture boils, turn down the heat to simmer on low heat for 5 to 10 minutes.
5. Remove from heat when the sauce is at the desired consistency.
6. Adjust seasoning to taste.

This is a good sauce for chicken or turkey. Just add the sauce during the last minutes of baking or grilling. It can also be used as a dipping sauce.

Thousand Island Salad Dressing

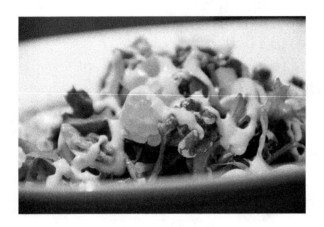

If you need a salad dressing, thousand island is popular on salads and as a sandwich spread. This adaptation makes the dressing keto-friendly for both purposes.

Prep & Cooking Time: 5 mins

Servings: 8 Servings
Nutrition Facts: Calories: 312 | Carbohydrates: 2g | Protein: 1g | Fat: 34g

Ingredients:

2 T olive oil
¼ c frozen spinach, thawed
2 T dried parsley
1 T dried dill
1 t onion powder
½ t salt

¼ t black pepper
1 c full-fat mayonnaise
¼ c full-fat sour cream
2 t lemon juice

Instructions:

1. Mix all ingredients in a small bowl.
2. Enjoy

This dressing can be covered and stored for up to 5 days.

Hollandaise Sauce

Since asparagus is a staple on keto diet plans, here is the traditional hollandaise sauce to accompany your spears. The sauce works on any vegetables. You will need to use a double-boiler for this sauce

Prep & Cooking Time: 25 mins

Servings: 4 Servings
Nutrition Facts: Calories: 566 | Carbohydrates: 1g | Protein: 3g | Fat: 62g

Ingredients:

4 egg yolks
2 T lemon juice

1 ½ sticks of butter, melted
salt and pepper

Instructions:

1. Heat water to boil in a saucepan.
2. Separate the eggs. Save the whites for another use.
3. Place the yolks in a heat-resistant bowl, either glass or stainless steel.
4. Carefully melt the butter in a saucepan without burning.
5. Place the bowl with the egg yolks over the simmering water to gently heat the eggs. Make sure the water is not touching the bottom of the bowl. The eggs need to be steamed, not cooked.
6. Add lemon juice to egg yolks.
7. Slowly stream the melted butter into the egg yolks while whisking. Start with a few drops of butter and then add a slow stream. Whisk the eggs the entire time until all the butter is added and the sauce has thickened.
8. Season to taste with lemon juice, salt, and pepper. You can also add a dash of tabasco sauce.
9. Serve over poached eggs or cooked vegetables.

Side Dishes

Mexican Cauliflower Rice

Give your cauliflower rice a spicy flair with this recipe. It's easy and quick and will be even faster using frozen cauliflower rice that has been thawed and drained in place of fresh.

Prep & Cooking Time: 25 mins

Servings: 8 Servings
Nutrition Facts: Calories: 90 | Carbohydrates: 4g | Protein: 3g | Fat: 8g

Ingredients:

1 head of cauliflower, riced
¼ c butter
⅓ c onion, minced
⅓ c tomatoes, diced
1 clove garlic, minced
¼ c jalapeño pepper, minced
1 T tomato paste
1 T chilli powder
½ t ground cumin
2 T lime juice
2 t olive oil
1 t salt
3 T fresh cilantro, chopped

¼ cup sharp cheddar cheese, optional

Instruction:

1. Wash cauliflower and grate to a texture resembling rice. This can also be done in a food processor. Set aside.
2. In a large skillet, heat pan to medium heat and melt butter. Sauté onion and garlic in the butter until soft.
3. Add tomatoes, jalapeño pepper, tomato paste, olive oil, chili powder, and cumin and stir until well mixed.
4. When the mixture in the pan is soft and fragrant, add riced cauliflower, lime juice, and salt.
5. Cook until riced cauliflower is the texture you prefer.
6. Top with fresh cilantro and cheddar cheese.
7. Serve while hot.

Green Beans and Bacon

This is a nice holiday side dish, but it can be a decadent dish for a regular day. It is fast and easy but tastes like it took hours to prepare. Combining bacon and a vegetable is also a good way to get non-vegetable eaters to give the green bean a try.

Prep & Cooking Time: 30 mins

Servings: 4 Servings
Nutrition Facts: Calories: 235 | Carbohydrates: 6g | Protein: 6g | Fat: 19g

Ingredients:

1 lb fresh green beans cut to 1" pieces
½ t salt
6 cloves garlic, minced
6 strips of raw bacon, chopped to ½ inch pieces

Instructions:

1. Boil green beans in water and salt to al dente. This should take about ten minutes.
2. Drain beans after they reach the desired texture and set aside.
3. In a large skillet, cook bacon until pieces are crisp.
4. Drain off all but 2 tablespoons of the bacon fat.

5. Add green beans into the pan with the bacon pieces and bacon fat.
6. Continue cooking green beans in bacon fat another 3 to 4 minutes until soft.
7. Add garlic and season with salt to taste.
8. Serve hot.

Baked Spaghetti Squash

Like pasta, but no pasta carbs. This can be a side dish that satisfies your carb cravings. Serve it as a side dish or add a protein and top with cheese to make it an entree.

Prep & Cooking Time: 45 mins

Servings: 4 Servings
Nutrition Facts: Calories: 31 | Carbohydrates: 7g | Protein: .6g | Fat: .6g

Ingredients:

1 spaghetti squash
1 T olive oil
1 t sea salt
1 t pepper

Instructions:

1. Preheat oven to 400 degrees.

2. Cut spaghetti squash in half lengthwise.
3. Set squash on cooking pan, cut side up.
4. Sprinkle olive oil, salt, and pepper over the squash halves.
5. Bake for 40 minutes until soft.
6. Remove squash from the oven and allow it to cool until it is easy to handle.
7. Scrape the squash out of the shell into a bowl.
8. Season with additional salt and pepper to taste.

This dish is easy to prepare and satisfying.

Snacks

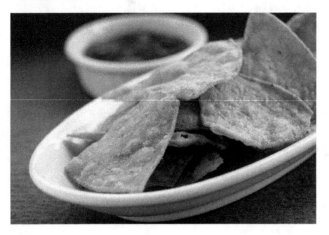

Taco Flavored Cheddar Crisps

Prep & Cooking Time: 15 mins

Servings: 6 Servings

Ingredients:

¾ c sharp cheddar cheese, finely shredded
¼ c parmesan cheese, finely shredded
¼ t chili powder
¼ t ground cumin

Instructions:

1. Preheat the oven to 400 degrees.
2. Line cookie sheet with parchment paper.

3. In a bowl, toss all ingredients together until well mixed.
4. Make 12 piles of cheese parchment paper.
5. Press down the cheese into a thin layer of cheese.
6. Bake for 5 minutes until cheese if bubby.
7. Allow to cool on parchment paper.
8. When completely cool, peel the paper away from the crisps.

These are a good keto substitute for chips. They are cheesy and crisp. Enjoy!

Keto Seed Crispy Crackers

With crackers being a pre-keto snack of the past, it is nice to be able to make a crispy cracker that can be served with cheese or spread with butter.

Prep & Cooking Time: 55 mins

Servings: 30 Servings of 1 cracker
Nutrition Facts: Calories: 61 | Carbohydrates: 1g | Protein: .2g | Fat: .6g

Ingredients:

1/3 cup almond flour
1/3 cup sunflower seed kernels

⅓ cup pumpkin seed kernels
⅓ cup flaxseed
⅓ cup chia seeds
1 tbsp ground psyllium husk powder
1 tsp salt
¼ cup melted coconut oil
1 cup boiling water

Instructions:

1. Preheat the oven to 300 degrees.
2. Stir all dry ingredients together in a medium-sized bowl until thoroughly mixed.
3. Add coconut oil and boiling water to dry ingredients and stir until all ingredients are mixed well.
4. On a flat surface, roll the dough between two pieces of parchment paper until approximately ⅛ inch thick.
5. Slide the dough, still between parchment paper onto a baking sheet.
6. Remove the top layer of parchment paper and place dough on a baking sheet into the oven.
7. Bake 40 minutes until golden brown.
8. Score the top of the dough into cracker sized pieces.
9. Leave in the oven to cool down.
10. When the big cracker is cool, break into pieces.

These crackers can be stored in an airtight container after they are completely cool.

Beef – Pork – Chicken

Slow Cooker Chilli

This chili is very tasty. The meat can be prepared ahead of time and transferred to the slow cooker when it's time to start cooking. Including celery gives the chili the texture missing without beans.

Prep & Cooking Time: 6 hrs 15 mins

Servings: 6 Servings
Nutrition Facts: Calories: 137 | Carbohydrates: 4.7g | Protein: 16g| Fat: 5g

Ingredients:

2 ½ lbs ground beef
1 red onion, diced
5 cloves garlic, minced
1 ½ c celery, diced
1 6-ounce can tomato paste
1 14.5 oz can diced tomatoes with green chilies

1 14.5 oz can stewed tomatoes
4 T chili powder
2 T ground cumin
2 t salt
1 t garlic powder

1 t onion powder

3 t cayenne pepper

1 t red pepper flakes

Instructions:

1. Cook ground beef in a large skillet.
2. Add onion, garlic, and celery and cook until ground beef browned
3. Drain the fat from the beef
4. Place beef and vegetable mixture into the slow cooker set on a low setting.
5. Add tomatoes and seasonings then stir to mix.
6. Place the lid on the slow cooker and cook on low for 6 hours.

Serve with cheese on top if desired. Adjust the red pepper to taste.

Chicken Parmesan

Chicken, sauce, and cheese make this low carb chicken dish delicious. It's easy to prepare so you can serve it even when you have a busy day. For a slightly less traditional, higher-fat version, use chicken thighs or boneless, skinless pork chops.

Prep & Cooking Time: 40 mins

Servings: 4 Servings
Nutrition Facts: Calories: 309 | Carbohydrates: 9g | Protein: 37g| Fat: 4g

Ingredients:

2 ¼ lb boneless skinless chicken breasts

1 T Italian seasoning
½ t onion powder
½ t salt
1 T olive oil
¼ c onion, chopped
4 cloves garlic, minced
1 bell pepper, diced
1 28 oz can crushed tomatoes
½ c shredded mozzarella
¼ c shredded parmesan

Instructions:

1. Preheat oven to 350 degrees.
2. Coat chicken breasts with Italian seasoning, onion powder, and salt
3. Heat skillet pan and add olive oil when hot.
4. Cook chicken, browning on each side until chicken is just done.
5. Remove chicken from pan and arrange in one layer in an oven-safe baking dish.
6. Using the same skillet as the chicken, cook onion, garlic, and bell pepper until soft.
7. Pour as much of can of tomatoes into the hot skillet as fits and stir until vegetables are incorporated into the tomatoes.
8. Pour any excess tomatoes over chicken, then pour the hot tomatoes sauce over the chicken.
9. Top with cheese.
10. Bake in preheated oven for 10-15 minutes until hot and bubbly and cheese is melted and golden brown.

If you need to sneak some low carb vegetables into the dish, add finely chopped raw spinach or broccoli into the sauce or sprinkle over the chicken before the sauce is poured.

Baked Un-BBQ Ribs

These ribs are proof you don't need a sugary sauce to enjoy ribs. The tangy flavor is from lime juice and lots of seasonings. You don't have to rely on packaged and bottled sauces and rubs to create a delicious pork centerpiece for your next meal.

Prep & Cooking Time: 1hrs 40 mins

Servings: 6 Servings
Nutrition Facts: Calories: 445 | Carbohydrates: 3g | Protein: 37g| Fat: 32g

Ingredients:

2 slabs baby back ribs
2 T olive oil
1 T garlic powder
1 t onion powder
1 t paprika
1 t salt
1 tsp cayenne pepper
Juice of 2 limes

Instructions:

1. Preheat oven to 350 degrees.
2. Remove membrane from the back of each slab of ribs.

3. Put remaining ingredients in a covered bottle or jar and shake well to mix.
4. Lay ribs on an aluminum foil-covered baking sheet, bone side down.
5. Pour seasonings over ribs, rubbing into the meat. Make sure both sides of both slabs get seasoning.
6. Reserve ¼ of the seasonings.
7. Flip ribs over every 30 minutes to brown both sides of the rib slabs.
8. About one hour into the cooking time, pour reserved seasonings over the top of the ribs.
9. Cook ribs until tender, should be about an hour and a half.

Season with salt and pepper as needed. This is a flavorful and enjoyable protein, worth saving your protein macros.

Fish

Salmon skewers

This recipe can be an appetizer or an entree. This is an easy, quick meal that is fun and interactive. We love to pick up our food and eat with our fingers. If prosciutto is unavailable, you can always use bacon.

Prep & Cooking Time: 30 mins

Servings: 4 Servings
Nutrition Facts: Calories: 680 | Carbohydrates: 1g | Protein: 28g| Fat: 62g

Ingredients:

¼ c fresh spinach, chopped fine
1 lb salmon cut into bite-sized pieces
¼ t black pepper, freshly ground
½ t pink Himalayan salt
1 T olive oil
3½ oz sliced prosciutto
1 c full-fat mayonnaise

8 wooden or metal skewers

Instructions:

1. Heat oven to 400 degrees.

2. Mix olive oil spinach salt and pepper in a 1-gallon storage bag.
3. Coat salmon pieces in oil mixture by placing them in the bag.
4. Place salmon on skewers.
5. Wrap salmon skewers with prosciutto.
6. Bake salmon for approximately 15 minutes turning every 3 or 4 minutes.
7. When prosciutto is crispy, and salmon is cooked, remove from oven.
8. Serve with mayonnaise on the side.

This dish is flavorful, and the prosciutto adds a smokiness to the salmon. Dress up the mayo with a teaspoon of garlic for extra zest.

Coconut Salmon with Napa Cabbage

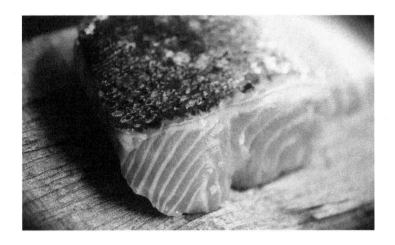

If you want to add an exotic flair to your salmon, try this recipe. The coconut and coconut oil give the dish a tropical feel. For a dipping sauce, try mixing Greek yogurt with turmeric and coconut cream. That will turn this delicious entree into finger food. Explore your exotic side with this salmon and Napa cabbage dish.

Prep & Cooking Time: 40 mins

Servings: 4 Servings
Nutrition Facts: Calories: 744 | Carbohydrates: 3g | Protein: 32g| Fat: 67g

Ingredients:

1¼ lbs salmon
1 T olive oil
½ c unsweetened shredded coconut
1 t turmeric
1 t kosher salt
½ t garlic powder
4 T olive oil, for frying
2 c Napa cabbage
1 stick butter
salt and pepper

Instructions:

1. Cut salmon into small 1-inch chunks.
2. Grind coconut to make it more likely to stay on the fish pieces. If you don't have a grinder, use a sharp knife to chop the shredded coconut as finely as possible.
3. Mix coconut, turmeric, salt, and garlic powder in a bowl.
4. In another bowl, coat salmon with 1 tablespoon of olive oil. Take
5. Dredge oil-coated salmon in dry ingredients.
6. Heat 4 tablespoons of olive oil in a frying pan to medium heat.
7. Cook coconut coated salmon until crispy. It will take about one minute per side. Make sure each side gets nicely browned.

8. Remove cooked salmon from the pan and keep warm while cooking the cabbage
9. Slice cabbage into thin strips with a knife or shred in a food processor.
10. Melt butter in pan used to cook salmon.
11. Cook cabbage until tender.
12. Season cabbage with salt and pepper.
13. Serve cabbage with salmon and enjoy.

Keto Tuna Casserole

If tuna casserole is one of your comfort dishes, this will be a keto version is a great way to satisfy tuna casserole needs. It is both economical and delicious, so a perfect fit if you are trying to do keto on a budget.

Prep & Cooking Time: 40 mins

Servings: 4 Servings
Nutrition Facts: Calories: 953 | Carbohydrates: 5g | Protein: 43g| Fat: 83g

Ingredients:

4 T butter
2 T olive oil
1 medium onion, diced
1 green bell pepper, diced
5 celery stalks, diced

2 c baby spinach chopped fine
2 large cans tuna in olive oil, drained
1 c mayonnaise
1 ½ c freshly shredded Parmesan cheese
1 t red pepper flakes
salt and pepper

Introduction:

1. Preheat oven to 350 degrees.
2. Heat butter and olive oil in a large skillet.
3. Sauté onions, green bell pepper, celery, and spinach in butter/oil.
4. In a bowl, mix tuna, Parmesan cheese, mayonnaise, and red pepper flake until thoroughly combined.
5. Add sautéed vegetables to the tuna mixture and stir until everything is incorporated
6. Pour tuna mixture into a casserole dish for baking.
7. Bake in the oven for 30 minutes.
8. Remove casserole from the oven when golden brown on top and bubbly.

This is a warm and comforting tuna dish that is quick to make. You can make the casserole the day before and store it in the refrigerator. Increase the baking time to 40 minutes when you put the cold casserole in the oven.

Vegetarian

Cinnamon Crunch Cereal

This is a vegetarian breakfast delight that is low in carbohydrates. It makes it easy to keep your protein macros in line when you need to eat less. This crispy sweet treat uses just a little stevia. You can adjust the sugar amount if necessary.

Prep & Cooking Time: 1 hr 40 mins

Servings: 6 Servings
Nutrition Facts: Calories: 129| Carbohydrates: 1g | Protein: 5g| Fat: 9g

Ingredients:

½ c flaxseed meal
½ c hemp seed meal
2 T ground cinnamon
½ t stevia
½ c water
1 T coconut oil

Instructions:

1. Preheat oven to 300 degrees.
2. Combine the dry ingredients (including stevia) in the bowl of a food processor.

3. Add water and coconut oil and mix until fully combined.
4. Add the apple juice and coconut oil and process until fully combined and mostly smooth.
5. Turn the batter onto a cookie sheet lined with parchment paper.
6. Spread it very thinly over the entire sheet.
7. Bake in the oven for 15 minutes.
8. After the 15 minutes are up, turn the heat down in the oven to 250 degrees.
9. Bake for an additional 5-7 minutes.
10. Remove the pan from the oven and cut the sheet of cereal into little squares. They should be small enough to fit on your spoon and eat.
11. Turn off the oven and put the cereal into the hot and cooling oven.
12. Leave in the oven for an hour,

This is a good cereal or snack. The recipe makes 6 ½ cup servings. It is so crunchy and delicious you will be tempted to snack throughout the day. This is good when you have used most of your macros but want a little something more.

Broccoli Cheese Fritters

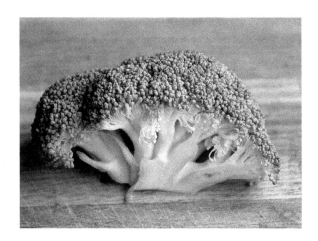

If you are a fan of corn fritters, these broccoli cheese fritters will be just what you are waiting for. Bursting with flavor, these morsels are

Prep & Cooking Time: 40 mins

Servings: 16 fritters w/sauce
Nutrition Facts: Calories: 104| Carbohydrates: 2g | Protein: 5g| Fat: 8g

Ingredients:

Fritters
¾ cup almond flour
7 T flaxseed meal
½ c fresh broccoli
½ c sharp cheddar cheese
2 large eggs

2 t baking powder
½ t hot sauce (without sugar)
Salt and Pepper to taste

Dipping Sauce
¼ c mayonnaise
¼ c cilantro, chopped
½ T lemon juice
Salt and pepper to taste

Instructions:

1. In a food processor, pulse broccoli until it is all in small uniform pieces.
2. In a separate bowl, mix almond flour, half of the flaxseed meal, and cheese.
3. Add eggs, hot sauce, and broccoli to the dry mixture and mix well.
4. Roll the batter into balls.
5. Put remaining flaxseed meal onto a plate.
6. Roll the batter ball in flaxseed meal to coat. Set on a plate or paper towel until fry time.
7. Heat up oil in a deep fat fryer to 375 degrees.
8. Put fritters on the basket and fry until brown. This will take from 3 to 5 minutes.
9. Fry in batches so there the basket is not crowded, and the fritters cook evenly.
10. Remove golden brown fritters from the fryer and drain on a rack with a paper towel underneath.
11. Season with salt and pepper.

12. Mix ingredients of dipping sauce in a bowl.

These fritters pair well with the dipping sauce. They are a nice keto-friendly addition to a meal or serve as snacks on game day. Finally, tailgating food that can be appreciated by everyone. They will not even realize the lack of cornmeal and white flour.

Asian Noodle Salad

This salad utilizes shirataki noodles, which are keto-friendly because they are mostly water. This makes a nice change while on a low-carb diet if you miss pasta. The Asian flavors are present in the salad and dressing. Eat it as an accompaniment to a meal or as an entire meal in itself. The flavor is fresh and delightful with all of the fresh vegetables, with Asian seasoning.

Prep & Cooking Time: 30 mins

Servings: 4 servings
Nutrition Facts: Calories: 212 | Carbohydrates: 6g | Protein: 7g| Fat: 16g

Ingredients:

Salad
1 c shredded red cabbage

1 c shredded green cabbage
¼ c scallions, chopped
⅓ c cilantro, chopped
4 c shirataki noodles, prepared and drained
¼ c chopped peanuts

Dressing
2 T garlic, minced
½ c water
1 T lime juice
1 T sesame oil
1 T gluten-free soy sauce
¼ c natural, unsweetened peanut butter
¼ t cayenne pepper
½ t salt
½ t stevia

Instructions:

1. Mix salad ingredients in a large bowl.
2. Place dressing ingredients in a blender and blend until smooth.
3. Pour dressing over salad and toss to coat salad with dressing completely.

This can be served room temperature or cold as a side dish or entree. Refrigerate any unused salad in an airtight container.

Dessert

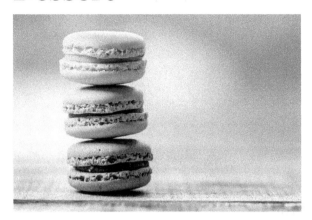

Cocoa Brownies

Like conventional brownies, all you need are the ingredients, and you can have brownies in an hour. The chocolate flavor comes through because there is so much of it. The sweetener tastes natural and a nearly flourless chocolate confection is created with only a few carbs. Thanks to the use of butter, the fat grams per browning are abundant.

Prep & Cooking Time: 40 mins

Servings: 9 servings
Nutrition Facts: Calories: 201 | Carbohydrates: 5g | Protein: 3g | Fat: 19g

Ingredients:

½ c salted butter, melted
1 c Granular Swerve Sweetener
2 Large Eggs
2 t vanilla extract
12 squares unsweetened baking chocolate, melted

2 T coconut flour
2 T cocoa powder
½ T baking powder
½ t salt
½ c walnuts, chopped (optional)

Instructions:

1. Preheat oven to 350 degrees.
2. Spray square baking pan with cooking spray or grease pan well with butter.
3. In a large mixing bowl, use an electric mixer or whisk and mix together butter and sweetener.
4. Add the eggs and vanilla extract to bowl and mix with an electric mixer for 1 minute until smooth.
5. Add melted chocolate and stir with a wooden spoon or spatula until the chocolate is incorporated into the butter mixture.
6. In a separate bowl, mix the dry ingredients (remaining ingredients besides walnuts) until combined.
7. Add dry ingredients into the bowl with the wet ingredients and stir with a wooden spoon until combined.

8. Add walnuts if desired.
9. Pour batter into prepared pan. Spread to cover the entire bottom of the pan and into corners.
10. Place in the center rack of the oven and bake for 30 minutes.
11. After the brownies are baked, take them out and leave them in the pan to cool.
12. When cool, cut them into 9 servings, and they are ready to eat.

These have to be a once-in-a-while treat because they are sweet, and if you're like me, that sugar will continue to call your name. These are so good you will have to work to eat only one serving.

Chocolate Chip Cookies

Chocolate cookies are a staple in most homes. You don't have to miss out just because you are on a low carbohydrate diet. These cookies will not be easily identifiable as low carb. That makes this a nice treat to share, so you aren't tempted to eat the entire batch.

Prep & Cooking Time: 30 mins

Servings: 24 cookies
Nutrition Facts: Calories: 120 | Carbohydrates: 3g | Protein: 2g | Fat: 11g

Ingredients:

1 ½ c almond flour
1 t baking powder
½ t salt
½ c butter, softened
½ c stevia
1 t vanilla extract
1 large egg
1 c sugar-free chocolate chips
½ c nuts, chopped

Instructions:

1. Preheat oven to 350 degrees.
2. Grease cookie sheets with butter and set aside.

3. In a large bowl, cream together the butter and the stevia.
4. Add the large egg and vanilla extract to the butter and stevia.
5. Mix until the egg is incorporated into the butter.
6. In a second bowl, mix together almond flour, baking powder, and salt until mixed well.
7. Add dry ingredients to the large bowl and mix until it is combined.
8. Add sugar-free chocolate chips and nuts and stir until they are distributed evenly.
9. Drop by spoonfuls onto the cookie sheet.
10. Bake until golden brown and the surface of cookies appear dry on the top and are cooked all the way through.
11. Remove cookies from sheet to a wire rack to cool.

Make these with or without nuts. Cocoa nibs can be used in place of the sugar-free chocolate chips. This is a good recipe to keep on hand so you can have a cookie along with everyone else. Make it a fun project with kids or friends. Baking is always a good way to bring people together, and this a recipe everyone will enjoy.

Keto Brown Butter Pralines

Quick and easy dessert with one net carb. Use a natural granulated sweetener like stevia to make the most of this recipe. There is some cooking, but no baking for these sweet tasty treats. Sprinkle with sea salt to add the salted caramel flavor that is so popular today.

Prep & Cooking Time: 16 mins

Servings: 10 servings
Nutrition Facts: Calories: 338 | Carbohydrates: 1g | Protein: 2g | Fat: 36g

Ingredients:

2 Sticks Salted butter
⅔ c heavy cream
⅔ c monk fruit sweetener
½ t xanthan gum
2 c pecans, chopped
Sea salt

Instructions:

1. Line a cookie sheet with parchment paper or use a silicone baking mat.
2. Prepare a cookie sheet with parchment paper or a silicone baking mat.

3. In a medium-size, medium weight saucepan, brown the butter until it smells nutty. Don't burn the butter. This will take about 5 minutes.
4. Stir in heavy cream, xanthan gum, and sweetener.
5. Take the pan off the heat and stir in the nuts.
6. Place pan in the refrigerator for an hour.
7. Stir the mixture occasionally while it is getting colder.
8. After an hour, scoop the mixture onto the cookie sheets and shape into cookies.
9. Sprinkle with sea salt.
10. Refrigerate on cookies sheet until the pralines are hard.
11. After the cookies are hard, transfer to an airtight container in the refrigerator.

This is a special treat. A low carb praline with the fat from the butter and cream. It is a nice dessert to have on a special occasion that you can work into your day without totally messing up your macros. The monk fruit sweetener is a 1:1 measure, so the texture is not altered by not using sugar. Give them a try and you will not be disappointed.

Conclusion

Thank you for making it through to the end of *Keto Diet for Women Over 50*, let's hope it was informative and able to provide you with all of the tools you need to achieve your goals in weight loss and a healthier lifestyle.

As women grow older, there are a variety of changes occurring within their bodies. Having a great deal of impact, the reduction of estrogen often causes weight gain and a slower metabolism. The keto diet, with adjustments for the particular requirements of women over fifty years old, is a wonderful way to lose weight while relieving some of the aches and pains experienced as the lack of estrogen takes hold. By adapting the diet to make it more palatable for women over the age of 50, the ketogenic diet can be beneficial in more ways than just weight loss. Follow the principals of food choices suggested by studies performed around the world and reap the benefits of this popular diet. Ease into ketosis with the plan outlined and you will find a smoother transition to a low-carbohydrate lifestyle. Use the tips and tricks given to smooth over rough spots and use the food list to try new foods.

You will have the most success on the keto diet by keeping track of your macros Maintain a record of the nutritional value of the foods you eat to avoid overeating. It can be easy to eat an excess of calories when putting an emphasis on eating fats. Eating a lot of meat makes it easy to eat an excess of protein. Failure to read labels can mean eating an unintended amount of carbohydrates. Take the time to learn what foods you like best and make plan your meals and snacks, so you stay on your macros. Make sure you eat lots of vegetable fiber and drink lots of water. The diet will work best when you to the time to count grams and calories.

You have the tools to be successful in losing weight on the keto diet. In the end, the weight loss will be the frosting on the. Don't worry; the cake will be made from almond flour and the frosting from stevia.

Finally, if you found this book useful in any way, a review on Amazon is always appreciated!

CPSIA information can be obtained
at www.ICGtesting.com
Printed in the USA
LVHW060741231220
674700LV00058B/94